Finding Your Emotional Balance

. . . .

 A JOHNS HOPKINS PRESS HEALTH BOOK

finding
your
emotional
balance

A Guide for Women

MERRY NOEL MILLER, MD

JOHNS HOPKINS UNIVERSITY PRESS

Baltimore

Note to the Reader: This book is not meant to substitute for medical care of people with emotional problems or mental disorders, and treatment should not be based solely on its contents. Instead, treatment must be developed in a dialogue between the individual and his or her physician. This book has been written to help with that dialogue.

Drug dosage: The author and publisher have made reasonable efforts to determine that the selection of drugs discussed in this text conform to the practices of the general medical community. The medications described do not necessarily have specific approval by the U.S. Food and Drug Administration for use in the diseases for which they are recommended. In view of ongoing research, changes in governmental regulation, and the constant flow of information relating to drug therapy and drug reactions, the reader is urged to check the package insert of each drug for any change in indications and dosage and for warnings and precautions. This is particularly important when the recommended agent is a new and/or infrequently used drug.

© 2015 Merry Noel Miller
All rights reserved. Published 2015
Printed in the United States of America on acid-free paper
9 8 7 6 5 4 3 2 1

Johns Hopkins University Press
2715 North Charles Street
Baltimore, Maryland 21218-4363
www.press.jhu.edu

Library of Congress Cataloging-in-Publication Data
Miller, Merry Noel.
  Finding your emotional balance : a guide for women / Merry Noel Miller, MD.
    pages cm. — (A Johns Hopkins Press health book)
  Includes bibliographical references and index.
  ISBN 978-1-4214-1833-9 (hardcover : alk. paper) — ISBN 1-4214-1833-9 (hardcover : alk. paper) — ISBN 978-1-4214-1834-6 (pbk. : alk. paper) — ISBN 1-4214-1834-7 (pbk. : alk. paper) — ISBN 978-1-4214-1835-3 (electronic) — ISBN 1-4214-1835-5 (electronic) 1. Depression in women. 2. Women—Health and hygiene—Popular works. I. Title.
  RC537.M545 2015
  616.85'270082—dc23   2015008452

A catalog record for this book is available from the British Library.

Special discounts are available for bulk purchases of this book. For more information, please contact Special Sales at 410-516-6936 or specialsales@press.jhu.edu.

Johns Hopkins University Press uses environmentally friendly book materials, including recycled text paper that is composed of at least 30 percent post-consumer waste, whenever possible.

CONTENTS

PREFACE

Being emotionally balanced means enjoying life when things are good and coping and recovering when bad things happen. An analogy might be sailing a ship: on a clear day it's smooth sailing, and in a storm-tossed sea you need sailing skills and reserves of strength to get through. We all need emotional balance in our lives, and yet it is so difficult for many people to find.

Women *and* men have emotional vulnerability throughout their lives. But this book is about women's emotional and mental health. We care about our appearance and worry about our weight, sometimes to our detriment when unhealthy eating behaviors consume us. We are twice as likely as men to become depressed. We seek help more often than men and seek to help others as well. We find ourselves trying to make everyone happy and take care of parents, spouses, and children. We try to do it all and sometimes doing it all is more than we can manage.

Starting at puberty, we experience hormonal cycles that influence our mood and can be hard to understand and hard to manage. Over time our bodies evolve, including, for many, the miracle of pregnancy and childbirth and the gradual changes that constitute menopause. Our psychology may be different from the psychology of men, and we may have a stronger need to feel connected to others.

How can we manage these many stages and phases of our lives? What are all the possible variations on "normal," and how can we know when our mood, our reactions, our behaviors are not normal? How can we protect ourselves from being overwhelmed? When should we seek help for ourselves? Where can we find help?

These are the questions I answer as best I can in this book. As a physician, psychiatrist, mother, wife, and daughter, I have spent my life discovering ways to achieve balance and helping others to do the same. This book shares the successful tools and tips that I have gathered both in my own life and through my work with patients over the past thirty years.

I focus my teaching and my medical practice on women's mental health, and I see the need for more resources to help women—resources that go beyond women's magazine articles by providing more detailed and specific suggestions. I have treated many women and have had the joy of seeing them recover. Some of these women are represented in these pages, although I have protected confidentiality by creating composites and changing the details. This book looks closely at the many challenges women face and guides you toward finding your own coping strategies and strength.

ACKNOWLEDGMENTS

I have many people to thank for their help in the preparation of this book. I have been fortunate to learn from many and to receive much support from family and friends during this process.

As I share in these pages, I have had my own personal struggles in life and have always dreamed of writing a book to share what I have learned both personally and professionally. After stepping down as chair of my department, I was given a sabbatical from my university for six months to begin writing this book. I am immensely grateful to many individuals who have helped me in this effort, and to East Tennessee State University for the gift of time for this project.

Thank you to the many patients who have trusted me to care for them. I incorporate some of your stories in this book (always taking care to conceal your identities).

Thank you to those who gave their time to read and give me feedback on the many drafts of this book as it evolved. Thank you to Katherine Cox and Carolyn Shamaya for painstaking editing of my early draft. I also greatly appreciate the input of Dr. Len Cruz, who gave my book a thoughtful review and made many suggestions. Thank you to Manjari Wijenake and to her daughter, Millie Wijenake-Bogle, for their helpful perspectives. Thank you also to Beth Begley, Elizabeth (Betty) Brown, Betty DeVault, Teresa Fletcher, JoAnn Foster, Dr. Paul Kelley, Dr. Jonathan Lipman, Njeru Muraguri, Dr. Greg Ordway, Beth Owen, Allyson Ross, and Joe Smith for their input.

Thank you to Jacqueline Wehmueller and to Johns Hopkins University Press for bringing this book to reality, and for much guidance and support.

My family has given me a lifetime of love and support. Thank you to my late father, Stanley Noel, my siblings Danny Noel and Melony Noel McKinnis, and my children, Drs. Corwin and Melanie Kay Miller. Thank you to my late husband, Dr. Barney Miller, who helped me tremendously to overcome my personal struggles and embrace life with joy. I especially appreciate the input of my husband, Gene Thune. He has been a great source of support throughout this process.

Finding Your Emotional Balance

The Who, What, and Why of This Book

Brenda is a physical therapist who has been very good at her job for many years. Recently a number of stressors have built up for Brenda, and she has become so depressed she is not able to work. She reluctantly came to see me for help, at the insistence of her husband. She hates her job now because she and other physical therapists have recently been criticized. She describes the job environment as hostile. She has also begun to doubt her ability to do the work, although she has always done it well in the past.

Brenda is also experiencing conflict with family members. Her brother, she says, is jealous of her and criticizes her often. Her mother often sides with her brother in family conflicts. She is raising a grandson with special needs because her son, who has a drug problem and no job, is unable to care for him. She has always spent a lot of time tending to others, but now feels she can no longer do it all. She feels overwhelmed easily, a big contrast with her previous ability to cope with stress. She cries, doesn't sleep well, has lost weight, and is having trouble concentrating. At times she wishes that she were dead.

I diagnosed Brenda as having major depression and started treating her with an antidepressant as well as psychotherapy. Brenda is deeply ashamed that she is depressed. She feels that it is a sign of weakness and she doesn't want others to know. She has been avoiding friends and condemning herself for being depressed. She has become more and more isolated.

Brenda shared with me that she had recently visited her primary care physician, and he was sorry to see her looking so down. He has treated her for years and also knows her as a colleague at the hospital. He views her as a competent and funny person. He shared with her that he, too, had experienced depression and that she should not be ashamed: it could happen to anyone. He urged her to stop blaming herself. She was grateful for his support and surprised to learn that he had been through similar struggles.

•

Any one of us may find ourselves in a situation like Brenda's. We may feel overwhelmed and need emotional support and professional assistance. But the stigma that surrounds mental illness often discourages people from seeking help. We live in a society that celebrates health, athletic success, good looks, and workplace performance. When a person is struggling with emotions, people can be unkind, sometimes even commenting on the individual's difficulty in functioning at his or her usual level. Often, acknowledging the need for emotional help is not easy.

I treat many patients with depression, and I tell them at their first appointment that I enjoy my job because I get to see people recover. I find it rewarding to help people who are in crisis, to help them regain their quality of life. Although psychiatric treatments are imperfect, much can be done to assist people whenever they have trouble in their life journey.

Much like Brenda's primary care doctor, I relate to my patients with depression very easily. I have experienced depression in my family and myself.

My Story

My own childhood experiences brought me to the field of psychiatry. I am the daughter of depression. My mother suffered from depression throughout the majority of my childhood. Her illness was a source of shame in my family. We were frightened and felt helpless as we watched her deteriorate. At times we were angry that she did not seem like other mothers. When I was growing up depression was not as well understood as it is today—the stigma was greater, and the treatments were less effective. My mother was given medications that caused her to gain significant weight and become lethargic. She spent her days lying on the couch. She went in and out of state psychiatric hospitals but did not improve. I was taught to keep her illness a secret and not to tell anyone what was wrong with her. My mother died of a heart attack when I was 18 years old, but really she had already lost her life years earlier due to depression.

Several years later, I became severely depressed while in medical school. Multiple stressors pushed me into despair, including a breakup with a boyfriend and the challenges of school. I felt the terror of losing my sense of self. I no longer recognized the person in the mirror. I felt unable to smile. I could not keep up with my studies and I took a leave of absence. I was terrified that I would never succeed in my goal of becoming a doctor but instead would sink into a life like my mother's.

I was much more fortunate than my mother. I found professional help and was given the time to heal, and I fully recovered. I had to start over in medical school but was able to successfully complete my education. I married, raised a family, and developed my career as a psychiatrist with no significant mood problems. I have enjoyed a full life with much joy. I joined a medical school psychiatry faculty and specialized in women's mental health issues in my clinical work, teaching, and research. I even was chosen to become chair of my department and served for over a decade.

More recently, I grieved deeply after the sudden death of my husband. We had been together for 32 years and were very happy. He died unexpectedly in his sleep. I was devastated by his death and fearful that this huge loss might lead me into depression again. I was determined not to succumb and instead used everything I had experienced and learned about mental health to help myself. I mourned my loss, but was able to regain my sense of joy over time. I learned about the grief process and gained personal and professional insights into the similarities and differences between grief and depression. I share these insights later in this book.

I can see now that in many ways my personal experiences with depression, grief, coping, and recovering have been the greatest gifts I've received. I developed a deep understanding, empathy, and passion for the field of psychiatry that has become part of my core and will never leave me. I acquired a sense of mission, a calling to do what I could to relieve the suffering of others. Together these experiences motivated me to write this book and share what I have learned. In the pages that follow I describe a wide array of emotional challenges for women, progressing through the life cycle from adolescence to life's later years. I hope that both my personal and professional experiences will be a help to others.

The Challenges Women Face

Throughout the life cycle, women face challenges. Some of these are challenges that both men and women face, and some are challenges faced only by women (just as men have their unique challenges, as well). There are many strategies that women can adopt to help them maintain balance, and a number of interventions are available to aid them when that balance is lost. As you read this book, you will see that a number of strategies are recommended for use during several life stages and for a variety of disorders. Indeed, there are some unifying concepts that can help all of us. For example, exercise and healthy nutrition are important for all ages and stages of life, for both physical and emotional health. I include nutritional recommendations throughout the book, because good nutrition can do so much to promote health.

An exciting development in psychiatry and medicine is the growing recognition of the link between physical health and emotional well-being. Thus we now understand better than ever that taking care of your body can help you take care of your mind as well. We have strong evidence, for example, that there is a clear relationship between depression and heart disease. People who have depression are at greater risk for developing heart disease, and people who have heart disease do worse if they are also depressed. Treating depression may help some people avoid heart disease or improve outcomes in people who have heart disease.

How This Book Is Organized

Part I follows a woman's life from adolescence to old age, discussing common problems and potential solutions at each phase of life. Within these chapters, I discuss specific mental disorders, such as depression, in the context of the life stage. An expanded discussion of these illnesses is found in the chapters making up part II of the book. Part II focuses on the major psychiatric illnesses that affect women and includes suggestions for preventing, identifying, and treating these conditions. I focus on illnesses that are more common or unique to women, or that pose special challenges for women.

Each chapter begins with stories portraying women who are dealing with the issues of that life stage or with a specific mental disorder. These stories are composites from my practice (except for one that is my own experience). The stories illustrate the problems that can occur in each life stage and each illness, and the rest of the chapter recommends specific suggestions for avoiding or managing problems. I discuss psychiatric treatments that are available, including types of therapy and medications. At the end of each chapter is a list of books, articles, websites, organizations, and support groups that you may find helpful. A bibliography at the end of the book identifies the professional references on which the text is based.

I hope this book will reach the hearts and minds of the many women and their family members who struggle with emotional issues. I hope it suggests ways of coping and encourages those who need professional help to reach out to get the help they need. You *can* find the resources you need, apply them to your situation, and restore your sense of joyful balance.

PART ONE

A WOMAN'S LIFE STAGES

CHAPTER 1

Navigating the Transition of Adolescence

Emily and her mother, Joan, were close until Emily became a teenager and the two of them began to clash. Emily was a good student who enjoyed a wide circle of friends. She liked hanging out with them, listening to music and talking. She was interested in a boy in her school and hoped they would start to date. Emily wanted to become more independent, and she began going to friends' houses without telling her mother. Emily saw no problem with this behavior since she had never been in trouble. Joan worried that Emily might fall in with the wrong crowd, and she tried to set limits on activities, especially on the weekends. Emily was annoyed that her mother was treating her "like a child." She wanted to make her own choices. Joan feared that Emily would begin drinking, using drugs, or engaging in sexual activity. Emily felt her mother did not understand her, and she started to confide primarily in her friends. The more Emily withdrew, the more her mother worried. When the two of them were together, their interaction was more and more conflicted, sometimes escalating to screaming matches. Joan missed the sweet days of Emily's childhood and thought she finally understood why other parents complained about the teenage years.

The Challenges of Adolescence

The transition from childhood to adulthood can be a difficult one. Many girls struggle with issues about their identity, self-esteem, relationships, body image, and mood. It can be overwhelming at times. Some girls become depressed, turn to alcohol or drugs, become self-destructive, or develop eating disorders. Others develop anxiety disorders (see chapter 7). This stage of life can seem tumultuous to both teenagers and their parents.

What is happening to girls during adolescence? For one thing, hormones start raging. Before puberty, levels of both estrogen and progesterone are stable and low, and girls are at no more risk for depression than boys. But everything changes with puberty, and from that point on girls are two to three times as likely as boys to experience depression.

Developmentally, adolescence is the time to establish yourself as a separate and independent person, no longer a child who is dependent on your parents. Teenagers may rebel and engage in acting-out behaviors during this period. Some start to defy their parents' rules. Some adolescents express their feelings of confusion and distress through self-destructive behavior, such as alcohol and drug use. Some experiment with cutting themselves. They often report feeling better after the cutting, as if there has been an emotional release.

Parents often feel challenged or even overwhelmed during their daughters' adolescence. Many parents struggle to find a way to maintain a positive relationship with their daughter who is changing before their eyes. The sweetness of childhood is often replaced by irritability and rebelliousness. Such changes are normal and expected, but that does not make them easy to endure.

Finding a way to guide your adolescent daughter through the rough waters of the teenage years requires a blend of nurturance and limit setting. Humor helps, too. You want to keep the lines of communication open but also be careful to maintain your position in your daughter's life as her mother, not her friend.

Sometimes mothers are tempted to lean on their daughters for emotional support, especially single mothers. Beware of this dynamic, since it can lead to an unhealthy shift in the relationship; your daughter may come to feel responsible for your well-being and feel neglected herself. Rather than turning to your daughter for support, it is healthier for you to turn to your own peers for advice and friendship. Be especially careful about venting to your daughter about your husband or ex-husband (whether or not he is her father). It may be tempting to talk to her about your marital issues, but she needs to maintain her own separate relationship with her father or stepfather and does not need to get pulled into ongoing conflict between married or divorced parents.

During the teen years, "acting out" behaviors can become problematic. Teens sometimes express their feelings or their distress nonverbally and become more uncooperative or oppositional. In extreme cases, adolescents may become openly defiant of authority figures such as their parents or teachers. In this situation, it may help for parents to take a step back and develop a concrete plan for expectations and consequences. To be most useful, rewards as well as punishments should be defined in advance. Clarifying expectations when everyone is calm with no immediate crisis can go a long way toward keeping emotions under control when acting out does occur.

This chapter focuses on three common concerns in adolescence: depression, eating disorders, and attention deficit disorder. Anxiety disorders may also occur at this age; these are discussed in depth in chapter 7. Whether you are an adolescent girl yourself or the mother of one, you may identify with some of these concerns and possible solutions.

Depression in Adolescence

Adolescence is a period of life when emotions may run high and setbacks may seem catastrophic. The teenager does not have the wisdom of age that she will later acquire and may feel devastated by losses. She is developing an inner world that is not easily accessible to others.

Depression has many causes (see chapter 6) and can affect people at any age. If you sense that you or your daughter may be becoming depressed, do not blame yourself. Depression is an illness that can happen to anyone. Some families are more vulnerable to depression due to their genetics—in looking at family members, it may be clear that a grandparent, a parent, an uncle or aunt, or a sibling suffered depression. Depression is an illness that can begin for no apparent reason—it can simply descend on a person. It also happens that stress, losses, and trauma can lead to depression or worsen it. In addition, negative, pessimistic thinking can contribute to depression, but then, too, depression can alter the thinking process so that the world seems more bleak and hopeless and events are interpreted more negatively.

Major depressive disorder can occur during adolescence, but symptoms may be different at this age than at other ages (see chapter 6 for a more complete description of the symptoms of depression). Depressed teens may not recognize that they are depressed or sad. Instead, their mood may be primarily irritable. They may argue more with others, especially their parents. Even adolescents who have always been cooperative in the past may be more easily angered by trivial slights.

Sleep and appetite can change for depressed adolescents, just as they can for adults. A young girl or teenager may have difficulty sleeping, or alternatively may sleep more than usual. Similarly, appetite can change in either direction—eating more or eating less. She may have difficulty concentrating and her performance at school may decline. She may be fatigued and have less energy and interest in her activities, and she may withdraw from friends and interests she enjoyed in the past.

Suicidal thoughts can occur at any age with depression. Self-destructive behaviors such as cutting may or may not be associated with the desire to die. Adolescents may turn to cutting themselves as a way to relieve their stress without consciously understanding why they are doing it.

When an adolescent has a setback, she may be more easily overwhelmed than an older woman experiencing the same obstacle. Adolescents who have losses, such as a breakup with a boyfriend or rejection by peers, may have difficulty trusting in the future and believing that they will feel better again.

If an adolescent makes a comment that sounds suicidal, the comment must be taken seriously. Suicide is the third leading cause of death for teenagers. A teenager is more at risk for suicide if she has depression, bipolar disorder, or an anxiety disorder, if she abuses drugs and/or alcohol, or if she has made previous suicide attempts. The risk increases if the adolescent is stressed and if the adolescent has access to firearms. Girls are more likely to attempt to harm themselves, and boys are more likely to complete suicide. But these numbers mean nothing, because girls do succeed in suicide. If you suspect that your adolescent loved one might be suicidal, you should ask her directly about her intentions: ask whether she has a specific plan and intends to act on her plan. Seek help for her if she indicates suicidal thinking. She may be angry with you in the short run but will likely be grateful in the long run if you get her into treatment promptly. Sometimes hospitalization is necessary. An assessment can be done by a professional if there is any question about her level of safety.

How to Distinguish Depression from an Eating Disorder

Many adolescents are slender, and there are numerous reasons why this is so. As girls' bodies change during the teenage years, it is common for them to become taller and thinner. Being thin runs in some families and is not necessarily a source of concern. On the other hand, a teen who loses weight or is significantly thinner than her ideal weight may have a problem. (Healthy weights according to height are standardized by medical experts and can be seen at websites such as cdc.gov, the website for the Centers for Disease Control and Prevention.)

Both depression and eating disorders can be associated with weight loss. If appetite decreases due to depression, a person can lose a significant amount of weight. This weight loss can easily be confused with the onset of an eating disorder. The key distinction is that in the case of an eating disorder, the girl or young woman thinks she is fat, and she is choosing not to eat for that reason. With depression, she may eat less because she is less hungry (although, as noted, some people with depression have an increase in their hunger).

The three primary eating disorders are anorexia nervosa, bulimia nervosa, and binge eating disorder. The first two generally begin during the teenage years, while binge eating disorder typically begins in adolescence or early adulthood but can start in later adulthood. Untreated eating disorders can create severe health problems, even death. They are serious illnesses.

An adolescent girl with *anorexia nervosa* (AN) may have the same appetite, but she will avoid eating because of her concerns about her weight. She may starve herself and also may purge (induce vomiting). She may or may not be willing to discuss her feelings about her weight with you, but she may make comments about herself to friends and family. She may develop significant health changes including loss of menstrual periods and osteoporosis. Her heart may be affected, which can be dangerous.

Bulimia nervosa (BN) is less easy to detect than anorexia nervosa, because it does not cause the person to lose weight. The primary symptom for this disorder is that these girls binge, or eat significantly more than is normal and healthy, and then eliminate the extra calories by making themselves vomit or by using laxatives and/or diuretics, exercising excessively, or alternating periods of bingeing with periods of starvation. The health problems caused by bulimia nervosa may be chronic and include impaired growth and digestive problems, tooth decay, and dangerous electrolyte imbalances such as low potassium levels.

The third main form of eating disorder is *binge eating disorder* (BED), in which bingeing occurs but is not followed by purging. As noted, binge eating disorder tends to begin later, with the average age of onset in the mid-twenties. Women who develop BED tend to gain weight and often develop obesity, with all of its medical consequences. Our nation is undergoing a surge in obesity, and often this problem begins in adolescence.

Girls who are developing an eating disorder are often secretive. They may not allow anyone to know what they are thinking and doing. Girls living with bulimia nervosa are often ashamed that they are purging and realize that other people would react negatively if they knew about it.

Another common feature of eating disorders is denial. Many girls with anorexia nervosa do not realize they have a problem. They see themselves as fat and are pleased as they lose weight, believing that others are wrong to be concerned about them. Girls with bulimia nervosa tend to be more aware that their behavior is not healthy and would not be acceptable to others, although they still may be reluctant to come forward for help.

Because of this secretiveness and denial, family members and friends, rather than the girl herself, may be the first to realize that something unhealthy is happening. These girls are not likely to come forward easily to ask for help.

Clues to the possible development of an eating disorder are:

- Changes in behavior around meals, such as wanting to eat alone and away from the rest of the family
- Development of rituals around eating, such as cutting food into little pieces
- Changes in dress, such as wearing multiple layers of baggy clothes, which may serve to hide the body as well as to preserve body heat (feeling cold is a problem for people who have anorexia nervosa)
- Moodiness and withdrawal (depression can occur in conjunction with the eating disorders)
- Disappearance to the bathroom after meals to purge
- Swelling of the cheeks due to inflammation of the glands after purging
- Erosion of the teeth

Eating disorders tend to evolve over time. A girl may begin to have some dissatisfaction with her body and start to experiment with restricting her diet and/or purging. If the process progresses, she may develop a full-blown eating disorder months or even years later. Reversing this process is much easier if it is caught early, so parents are wise to be alert for possible warning signs.

The largest group with eating disorders is composed of all the girls who have some of the symptoms or are starting to experiment with disordered eating behaviors but do not yet have the full-blown disorder. Technically these girls are diagnosed as having other specified feeding or eating disorder (OSFED) in our diagnostic system. These girls may be dieting excessively or bingeing or purging occasionally and are at considerable risk to progress to the full-blown disorder. Early intervention is key.

Although I have described the separate eating disorders as distinct conditions, in reality there is much fluidity between them. For example, a girl may start to develop anorexia nervosa early in her teens and evolve to have bulimia nervosa at age 20. She may improve, and then have a recurrence of the disorder at a point later in her life when she is under stress.

Depression and eating disorders can certainly exist together. About half of girls with anorexia nervosa and half of girls with bulimia nervosa develop depression. It is important to know about this coexistence and to look for it. The treatments for depression are different from those for eating disorders, and treatment can only be optimal if both disorders are identified and treated if they are occurring together. Both conditions have significant risks.

Recognizing Attention Deficit Disorder in Girls

Attention deficit disorder (ADD) and *attention deficit hyperactivity disorder* (ADHD) are problems that sometimes first develop in childhood or adolescence. Although ADD and especially the hyperactivity of ADHD are more common in males, they can occur in females as well.

The symptoms of ADD are:

- Failure to pay close attention to details, or the tendency to make careless mistakes, such as in schoolwork
- Difficulty sustaining attention and remaining focused
- Often not seeming to listen when spoken to directly

- Failure to follow through on instructions and to finish schoolwork, chores, or other duties; being easily side-tracked, failing to finish tasks, shifting instead from one uncompleted task to another
- Difficulty organizing tasks and activities
- Avoidance of tasks that require sustained mental effort, such as homework
- Often losing things needed for tasks and activities (books, homework, eyeglasses, cell phone)
- Being easily distracted by outside stimuli and unrelated thoughts
- Being frequently forgetful in daily activities (doing chores, running errands)

Hyperactivity is added to the attention deficit symptoms when a person has ADHD. The signs of hyperactivity are:

- Fidgeting
- Difficulty sitting still
- Feeling restless or running about
- Difficulty playing or engaging in leisure activities quietly
- Feeling often "on the go," restless, or difficult to keep up with
- Often talking excessively
- Often blurting out an answer before a question is completed
- Difficulty waiting one's turn
- Often interrupting or interfering with others

Many girls who have ADD are not diagnosed, especially since inattention is less noticeable to others compared to hyperactivity. The lack of diagnosis may lead the girl to develop low self-esteem as she experiences repeated failures at home, school, and elsewhere. She is likely to have poor grades and to think of herself as "bad" because she is often unable to control her impulses. She may engage in high-risk behaviors such as substance abuse. She may develop depression along with ADD.

If you suspect that you or your daughter may have ADD or ADHD, you should seek an evaluation. Information and observations from parents and teachers are frequently helpful in making the diagnosis. A number of treatments can be effective, including medications and behavioral therapies. Stimulants have the paradoxical effect of helping those who have true ADD to be calmer and more focused, but many of them are addictive and must be used with caution. Some medications used for ADD are also abused, so prescription drugs should be carefully guarded and monitored. The combination of therapy and medications may be very helpful for getting back on track for those who have ADD or ADHD.

Finding Help: What to Do If You Have an Eating Disorder

ACKNOWLEDGE THAT IT EXISTS

Right off you should know that eating disorders are dangerous and are not to be ignored. The first step in addressing a possible eating disorder is to acknowledge that it exists. This is often the most difficult step since girls frequently do not want to admit to themselves or anyone else that they are deliberately restricting their diet, bingeing, and/or purging. If you are a girl who realizes she is getting into unhealthy behaviors with eating, you need to get help.

GET HELP

- Find a way to talk to a concerned family member or school counselor. Expect that it will be hard, but do not give up.
- Get a medical evaluation to detect possible health complications. Eating disorders can be fatal, as we see in the dramatic news stories that appear from time to time about the death of a model or celebrity who has an eating disorder. You need to have blood work and an overall physical examination done. If you have anorexia nervosa, you may also need a bone scan to determine if your bones have been weakened and made vulnerable to fractures.

- Seek an individual therapist who has experience with adolescents with eating disorders. Therapy is the mainstay of treatment and it is important to find someone with whom you feel rapport. Expect that it will take time to make changes.
- Consider family therapy in conjunction with individual therapy. Family therapy has been shown to be effective for the treatment of anorexia nervosa in adolescents. In particular, the "Maudsley method" has been demonstrated in several studies to be more effective for adolescents than individual therapy alone. This method was created at the Maudsley Hospital in London and includes the parents in the treatment process in a central way. In this approach, parents are empowered to participate in the refeeding process for their daughter until she restores her weight to an adequate level. Control is an important issue for adolescents, especially those with anorexia nervosa, and parents are encouraged to hand control back to their daughters as they achieve their weight goals.
- Seek the advice of a nutritionist or another professional to analyze your diet and plan foods that you consider "safe" as well as to maintain adequate nutrition. If you have bulimia nervosa or binge eating disorder, a nutritionist can help plan your daily meals in an effort to eat at frequent intervals and not allow yourself to get too hungry, which can lead to bingeing. Often BN turns into a vicious cycle in which someone tries to diet, gets very hungry, eats more than she means to eat, purges, and then sometimes has a feeling of relief. Other factors may also trigger a binge, such as boredom or loneliness. Planning ahead for how you are going to eat each day can make you less vulnerable to bingeing and then purging, and can turn the vicious cycle around.
- Consider seeing a psychiatrist for an evaluation, preferably someone with experience treating people who have eating disorders. A psychiatrist may prescribe medication,

such as an SSRI (see chapter 6), which can reduce bingeing and purging.
• Look into specialized eating disorder programs. If the above combination of outpatient approaches is not successful, or if your symptoms are very severe, you may need treatment at a specialized eating disorder program. There are programs around the country with this focus. Some are at hospitals, some are at residential facilities, and some are intensive outpatient programs. You can get more information on these programs as well as other information on eating disorders at the websites listed below for the National Eating Disorders Association and for the Eating Disorders Coalition.

How Mothers Can Help Adolescent Daughters with Their Moods

OPEN COMMUNICATION IS KEY

• Help your daughter feel safe to tell you what is happening in her life. Provide opportunities for her to confide in you.
• Be watchful for signs of changed behavior. Be alert for any signs of suicidal thinking in a depressed teen, and do not be afraid to ask about it.
• Pay attention to the cycling of her mood. With the onset of menstruation girls become susceptible to premenstrual syndromes (see the next chapter). Simply becoming aware of this cycling can help you both to understand what is happening if she becomes more moody.
• Set clear limits and identify consequences for behavior problems. Although adolescents crave freedom and independence, they need structure and guidance from their parents. Clarify what is expected of her (such as her curfew and chores), and spell out the penalties for "acting out." Establish an understanding of these expectations at a calm time, rather than in the heat of a dispute.

ENCOURAGE HEALTHY ACTIVITIES

- Urge her to be physically active and to get involved in sports or special-interest clubs and other groups. Also encourage her to read books and to make the most of her academic pursuits. These activities can boost her self-esteem and protect her mood.
- Encourage supportive close friendships, especially if she is not inclined to join groups.
- Commend efforts that she makes that are healthy. Help her to develop beneficial lifestyle habits, including getting enough sleep and eating a well-balanced diet.
- Keep nutritious food in the house.
- Be cautious about commenting on her weight. By the same token, avoid making comments about your own weight and the weight of other women. Help her to avoid prioritizing weight over her other attributes.

SEEK PROFESSIONAL RESOURCES

- Pursue resources for therapy if it is needed. A variety of professionals may be able to provide therapy, including social workers, psychologists, and psychiatrists. A school counselor may also be helpful. Through therapy, your teen can learn to express her feelings and gain insight about her behavior.
- Consider including all members of the household in family therapy in addition to individual therapy for the teen. Including family members in therapy has the potential to improve communication patterns now and for the future, and increase support for the teen.
- Discuss the possible need for contraceptives if she is sexually active. This is a delicate topic and may be best discussed between the teenager and her primary care physician.
- Consider medication. If your daughter is depressed, selective serotonin reuptake inhibitor (SSRI) antidepressants

may be recommended (ideally in conjunction with therapy). Be aware that there is a warning from the Federal Drug Administration (FDA) about a possible increase in suicidal thoughts in adolescents who are prescribed SSRIs. This warning is based on limited data that suggested a very small risk: a study of 2,000 children treated with either an SSRI or placebo found that 4 of the adolescents taking an SSRI developed suicidal thoughts compared to 2 of the adolescents taking a placebo. None of the adolescents in that study made an attempt, and other studies have been unable to replicate this finding. Suicidal thinking can occur due to depression itself. SSRI antidepressants may have much benefit, and may prevent suicide in depressed teens.

• Remember that your daughter's depression is not her fault and it is not your fault! Seek to help her, but do not assume that you are to blame.

How You Can Get Help for Low Mood If You Are an Adolescent Girl

BE SURE TO TALK WITH SOMEONE ABOUT HOW YOU ARE FEELING

• If you develop suicidal thoughts at any time, it is essential that you tell a trusted adult. Talk to your parents, school counselor, therapist, or doctor.

• If you are feeling down, consider talking to someone about what you are experiencing. You could start with a friend or your mother, or perhaps a school counselor. There are probably more people around who could help than you realize.

• Get in touch with your mood. Writing in a journal or diary may help you make sense of how you are feeling. Learn to give yourself the advice that you might give to a friend. It may benefit you to write down several good things that have happened each day.

- Pay attention to the timing of your moods. Are you more likely to feel down before your menstrual period? That could suggest a premenstrual problem (see chapter 2). Do you feel more anxious and down before meals, when you are hungry? That might suggest that your blood sugar is low and you need to eat more regularly. Is it hard for you to be alone? That might be something for you to work on as a goal as you grow older.

STAY ACTIVE AND HEALTHY

- Exercise is terrific for improving your mood. If you're not in the habit of keeping fit, start with walking, or any sport that you enjoy. You will likely find that you feel calmer and less stressed afterward.
- Keep in mind that you should avoid alcohol and drugs. They may seem like a way to help your mood improve, but in the long run they will likely make you feel more down.
- Try to eat healthy food and get enough sleep.

TAKE ADVANTAGE OF THE HELP OFFERED BY PROFESSIONALS

If you try all these strategies and your low mood persists, you may have a clinical depression.

- See a therapist or counselor. Ask your parents or another trusted adult, such as the school counselor, to arrange for you to see a therapist. A therapist can be a social worker or a psychologist or a psychiatrist or another professional who is trained to do therapy (such as a marriage and family counselor). In therapy sessions you will have a safe place to freely and privately discuss your feelings with a professional who is trained to help you.
- Involve your family. In addition to going to individual therapy, you might find it useful to participate in family therapy, where other family members see a therapist with

you. If there are family issues that are playing a role in why you are feeling low, consider this: getting to the heart of the matter may require including other individuals in your life.

- Consider medication if it is recommended. If you continue to have symptoms of depression after being in therapy, you may benefit from an evaluation for an antidepressant medication. Your therapist and/or parents can help find someone for you to see who can prescribe this kind of medication. This type of medication is not addictive and has the potential to improve the symptoms of depression that may be plaguing you. Sleep, appetite, energy, concentration, interests, and motivation are all likely to improve with the right choice of medication.
- Do not feel ashamed if you need help. Many people experience depression, and you can feel better.

•

Adolescence is a time of life when many changes are occurring, and emotions commonly become more volatile. The hormonal changes of adolescence can make it hard to know what is "normal" and what is not. It is common to have mood swings to some extent, and for girls to start to pull away from their parents in order to become more independent. However, some girls develop depression, anxiety, substance abuse, eating disorders, attention deficit disorder, or other problems. Refer to chapters 6, 7, and 8 for more detailed information on depression, anxiety, and substance abuse. The good news is that help is available.

For parents, adolescence can be frightening and exasperating. I have been told that adolescence may be "God's way of helping parents let go of their children." Know that these sometimes-tumultuous years are a stage that will not last forever. If you can both navigate this period successfully, you and your child can emerge with a healthy adult relationship in the future.

RECOMMENDED RESOURCES

BOOKS

Francis Mark Mondimore, MD, and Patrick Kelly, MD. *Adolescent Depression: A Guide for Parents*, second edition. Baltimore: Johns Hopkins University Press, 2015.

Gerald D. Oster, PhD, and Sarah Montgomery, MSW. *Helping Your Depressed Teenager: A Guide for Parents and Caregivers*. New York: John Wiley & Sons, 1995.

Lisa Schab, LCSW. *Beyond the Blues: A Workbook to Help Teens Overcome Depression*. Oakland, CA: Instant Help Books, A Division of Harbinger Publications, 2008.

Deborah Serani, PsyD. *Depression and Your Child: A Guide for Parents and Caregivers*. Lanham, MD: Rowman & Littlefield, 2013.

WEBSITES

For fighting alcohol and drug abuse: www.drugfree.org/resources

For helping girls bond: www.opheliaproject.org

For information on eating disorders: www.nationaleatingdisorders.org and www.eatingdisorderscoalition.org

CHAPTER 2

The Spectrum of Premenstrual Disorders

Susan came to see me ten years ago because every month she was having mood problems, especially irritability, just before her menstrual period. She described being overwhelmed by her job as a schoolteacher at that time of the month, easily annoyed by her students. She received a complaint from her principal that she had been heard yelling at her class, and she was worried she could lose her job. She found it difficult to interact with her husband and manage her own children. Her mood improved each month once her menstrual period began. Her symptoms varied from month to month, some months severe and some months not so bad. Occasionally her symptoms were so severe that she would stay home from work.

My first recommendation to Susan was that she should start charting her moods to verify that her symptoms occurred primarily when she was premenstrual. I also recommended that she exercise. Susan continued to have severe premenstrual symptoms. Her charting revealed that she had depression throughout the month, and that her depression worsened premenstrually. I started her on fluoxetine (Prozac) at a constant daily dose and asked her to continue charting. Her depression showed improvement within the first month, but Susan reported that she continued to have "breakthrough" symptoms of irritability when she was premenstrual. After several months of this pattern, we decided to adapt her dosing regimen, so she took an additional small dose of fluoxetine for the week before her period was expected. She was happy to tell me at her next visit that her moods had leveled out.

What Is PMS? Is It Real?

Premenstrual Syndrome (PMS) is a topic that has been the subject of ridicule, controversy, and scholarly debate. Few medical disorders rival PMS as a target of humor. A host of conflicting theories about possible causes, and many unproven remedies, have been promoted. Because physicians aren't able to identify the cause of PMS or offer reliable treatments for it, the public remains confused and skeptical that it even exists.

Can you think of any illness that receives as much scorn as PMS? The chameleon-like nature of women with PMS, and in particular their tendency to be irritable and oversensitive, has led to a good bit of ribbing and derision. Over the years I have acquired a number of coffee mugs, bumper stickers, and calendars with jokes on this topic. It seems unusual for an illness to provide material for jokey bumper stickers, right? This emotional problem is easily minimized and mocked, and one possible reason for this is the broad range of symptoms and severity. Because many women have mild levels of symptoms, it is easy to think that the problem is not a genuine one. Most of us would not make fun of someone with a truly serious disorder, but PMS has not been widely viewed as significant, and its legitimacy has often been questioned. Is PMS important? Is it really an illness?

Women who see their doctors for help with psychiatric symptoms that are related to the menstrual cycle often "fall through the cracks." Traditionally psychiatry departments have taught their students little about the menstrual cycle, and gynecologists have limited training or time for focusing on emotional or behavioral symptoms. Some doctors and lay people have openly doubted whether such a syndrome exists and have given little attention to learning how to help women with symptoms. Furthermore, because of the variability of the menstrual cycle, researchers have excluded women from many drug studies. It is simpler to look for potential benefits of medications by studying the effect on men who do not have this additional "variable" of monthly changes in mood, rather than seeing menstrual variation itself as a legitimate subject of study.

Controversy has swirled around this diagnostic entity. Although premenstrual symptoms have been observed and described for thousands of years, the medical field has only recently accepted PMS as a legitimate illness. Why is there so much debate?

Premenstrual Disorders

What the general public knows as PMS encompasses several different conditions, a whole spectrum of disorders. Premenstrual symptoms may range in severity from mild discomfort, to the commonly recognized PMS, to the newly defined psychiatric disorder premenstrual dysphoric disorder (PMDD). And there are also women who experience premenstrual exacerbation of another disorder (PME), which means that the symptoms of their disorder get worse around the time of their period.

Premenstrual symptoms are extremely common, with as many as 95 percent of women affected by at least one symptom during their childbearing years. These premenstrual changes may be mild—and for the vast majority of women are not disabling and are of little concern.

Approximately 30 to 50 percent of women experience two or three premenstrual symptoms without enough severity to interfere with functioning. These women may be said to have PMS, and they rarely seek medical consultation for this problem. They may choose to use over-the-counter (OTC) medications and may mention these symptoms at routine gynecological examinations.

Only about 3 to 5 percent of women experience premenstrual symptoms that are severe enough to interfere with functioning and to qualify for the diagnosis of PMDD. This diagnosis requires the presence of five or more symptoms, one of which must involve mood, which are severe enough to impair daily functioning (either social or occupational). Mood symptoms can include depressed mood, irritability, anxiety, and mood swings.

Note that timing is key to the diagnosis of PMS and PMDD: symptoms must occur during the seven to ten days prior to onset of menses and resolve within a few days after menses begin. Precise knowledge of the timing of symptoms within the menstrual cycle is critical to accurate diagnosis, and therein lies a big problem with both the research that has been done on PMS and the clinical evaluation of women who have PMS. When women are asked after the fact about their symptoms (called "retrospective memories") and when in the menstrual cycle symptoms occurred, their recollections have been shown to be highly inaccurate. The only truly valid way to assess for PMS and PMDD is to have patients record their symptoms daily, "in real time." Many studies in the past have failed to track symptoms, and their results are questionable.

In short, three elements are key to making the diagnosis of PMDD: (1) Timing of the appearance and disappearance of clinical symptoms; (2) evidence of significant impairment of work, social activities, or relationships with others; and (3) evidence that the symptoms are not merely worsening of the symptoms of another disorder. PMDD can potentially cause 1,400 to 2,800 symptomatic days in the course of a woman's reproductive years, which is equivalent to three to eight years' worth of symptoms.

Premenstrual symptoms experienced by women vary greatly. In fact, over 150 different symptoms have been identified in association with the premenstrual period. The most common psychological symptoms include depressed mood, anxiety, mood swings, flashes of anger and irritability, loss of pleasure, and the sense of loss of control. A number of physical symptoms can occur as well, including abdominal bloating, breast pain, headache, flu-like symptoms, increased appetite and cravings (especially for sweet and salty foods), and changes in sleep pattern.

Many women who see their doctors for evaluation of what they perceive to be PMS will be found, upon closer evaluation, to have symptoms throughout the month that worsen when they are premenstrual. When this phenomenon occurs, patients may be said to have premenstrual exacerbation of another disorder. The most common disorder that has been found in women with PMS is major depression: in fact, as many as 50 percent of women who report that they have PMS have been found to have major depression with premenstrual exacerbation.

A number of other disorders may also demonstrate premenstrual exacerbation in a subset of female patients. These include both psychiatric and medical conditions. Some patients with panic disorder, for example, will report increased incidence and severity of panic attacks when they are premenstrual. The same is true for the symptoms of a number of other conditions: generalized anxiety, post-traumatic stress disorder (PTSD), obsessive-compulsive disorder (OCD), bulimia nervosa, substance abuse, mania, and psychosis.

Patterns of Premenstrual Syndromes

PMS and its variants may begin any time from puberty to menopause, but women seeking treatment are most often in their thirties. Typically, symptoms worsen with age until menopause. Women with a history of premenstrual disorders may also be at risk for mood symptoms if they take hormonal therapy for menopause, especially if they take progesterone. Women who have had hysterectomies without removal of their ovaries may continue to experience symptoms, although the severity may be lessened. Abdominal pain or pelvic pain is not characteristic of a premenstrual disorder and suggests possible *endometriosis*, which is a condition where uterine tissue is found outside the uterine lining and undergoes changes during the menstrual cycle. Premenstrual disorders should be clearly distinguished from *dysmenorrhea*, which is pelvic pain that occurs during menstruation, not before.

Premenstrual disorders show no clear association with socioeconomic status and have been observed in women all over the world. Some cultural variability has been described in the nature and severity of specific symptoms: for example, fewer Japanese women have breast symptoms; Nigerians more often report headache; and American women more often report irritability.

Much evidence suggests a link between PMDD and the mood disorders. Both disorders show a significant family history of depression. The presence of PMDD increases a woman's risk for developing a future episode of major depression. As mentioned previously, major depression may worsen premenstrually, and a woman is more likely to be depressed enough to visit the emergency room and to be admitted to the hospital when she is in the premenstrual phase.

The onset and duration of premenstrual symptoms within a monthly cycle may vary greatly. Symptoms may occur at ovulation and then recur when a woman is premenstrual, or may begin at ovulation and gradually increase until the period begins, or may only occur shortly before menstruation. Severity can also vary greatly from month to month.

What Is the Social Impact of PMS?

PMS has been recorded since the time of Hippocrates, who described women having headaches and a sense of heaviness. Socially and legally, the diagnosis of PMS has been used both to discriminate against women and as a rationale to give them special consideration. PMS has been used in the legal arena as far back as 1845, when a maid was acquitted of the charge of murdering her employer's child on the grounds of insanity due to "obstructed menstruation." In the 1950s, PMS received more legal attention as questions were raised about the criminal and civil responsibility of women who had automobile accidents during their premenstrual phase. Several highly publicized criminal trials involving PMS as a defense have occurred abroad since the 1980s: in particular, three women who had PMS symptoms were successful in their pleas for diminished responsibility or mitigating circumstances to their charges of manslaughter, arson, and assault. The successful employment of PMS as a defense led to widespread debate about the validity of this diagnosis and its use as a reasonable argument.

Many have debated the legitimacy of this diagnostic category. It is no wonder there has been controversy about PMS: at the one extreme are those who question its existence, and at the other extreme are those who successfully argue that it lessens responsibility for murder! It is only in the most recent revision of the American Psychiatric Association's diagnostic manual, the *Diagnostic and Statistical Manual of Mental Disorders* (DSM-5, 2013), that PMDD has been recognized and considered an official category. After considerable and contentious review, this diagnosis has been accepted within psychiatry.

What Causes Premenstrual Syndromes?

Many theories have been advanced about possible causes of PMS and PMDD, which has led to a wide variety of treatment approaches (described below). The evidence for most of these theories is weak, and overall the cause of PMS remains unclear. Although it seems intuitive to assume that the hormonal changes that occur within the menstrual cycle must cause the symptoms of PMS, the evidence suggests that the cause of PMS is more complex. More likely, hormones interact with other regulatory systems to create this syndrome.

Many studies have tried to identify abnormal hormone levels during the premenstrual phase or to correlate symptom severity with changes in hormone levels. However, these efforts have generally failed to demonstrate any consistent pattern. There is no hormonal abnormality that can be measured, and there is no reason to obtain hormonal levels in women with premenstrual symptoms. Hormone levels would not tell you anything helpful regarding whether you have this disorder. Since there is no diagnostic test for PMS, the diagnosis is based on history.

How Can PMS or PMDD Be Distinguished from Bipolar Disorder?

Mood swings are a symptom of several conditions. We have been discussing PMS and PMDD in this chapter, but bipolar disorder is another condition in which moods fluctuate widely. A person with bipolar disorder can experience extended periods of depression and other times with days to weeks of elation or irritability (see chapter 11). Mood changes for women with bipolar disorder are not necessarily linked to the menstrual cycle, but a woman with bipolar disorder might also have PMS or PMDD, in which case her symptoms may be more severe when she is premenstrual. For example, she may have premenstrual worsening of depression or mania. It can be hard to tell if a woman has PMS/PMDD, bipolar disorder, or both. Charting symptoms on a calendar generally helps women recognize whether their mood is related to their menstrual cycle.

What Can You Do If You Have Premenstrual Disorder?

Treatment strategies depend on the severity of the symptoms. I will list approaches that *may* work, but there is limited evidence of the effectiveness of some therapies. Along with each treatment I will summarize what medical research has shown about its efficacy.

CHART YOUR MOOD THROUGHOUT THE MONTH

- See the big picture. If you suspect you have PMS or PMDD, start charting your mood symptoms on a calendar throughout the month. You can also use a PMS tracker chart to keep a record of your moods (see figure 1). Day one refers to the day that your period begins. Only by looking at a diary of your symptoms can your doctor know if you have PMS. As mentioned previously, about half of all women who think that their symptoms are premenstrual find, by charting symptoms, that they have the symptoms throughout the month, with some worsening premenstrually.

• Look for patterns. In addition to clarifying whether you have PMS, charting your mood can itself be therapeutic by giving you better insight into your body, more of a sense of control. You can also look for patterns that might help you to understand your mood changes. Depending on the severity of your symptoms, you may choose to plan some of your activities around the days when you predict more difficulty.

CHANGE YOUR DIET

• Limit carbohydrates. Many women who have PMS develop carbohydrate craving during the premenstrual week. Similar appetite disturbances may be observed in several other disorders: seasonal affective disorder, binge eating disorder, and bulimia nervosa. In women with these disorders, evidence suggests that the consumption of simple carbohydrates may elevate mood temporarily, but that overeating carbohydrates may unintentionally create a vicious cycle in which temporary relief is followed by increased feelings of fatigue and depression. Several studies suggest that some women achieve a more permanent control of their mood by eliminating simple carbohydrates from their diet, especially refined sugar: for example, by avoiding candy, table sugar, packaged cereals, and cake.

• Eat smaller, frequent meals. It is strongly recommended that women with mood problems eat several small meals a day rather than one or two large ones and that they favor complex carbohydrates (such as pasta and whole wheat bread) and protein.

• Eliminate caffeine. Eliminating caffeine products (such as coffee, tea, and some sodas) can help control your moods and is often recommended for women with PMS and PMDD.

Not only does caffeine affect mood in women with PMS but it also may be metabolized more slowly in this group than in other women or men, so the caffeine ingested has a longer and larger effect. Also, reducing caffeine may help with moods in general.

• Reduce salt. Women are often advised to reduce salt intake to lessen PMS swelling, breast tenderness, and abdominal bloating. However, lowering salt intake has not been shown to relieve the mood symptoms of PMS.

• Avoid alcohol. As is commonly recommended, avoid alcohol if you have PMS or PMDD. Women with PMS have been shown to drink significantly more alcohol overall, but this increase is not limited to the premenstrual period and instead occurs throughout the month.

TAKE VITAMINS AND NUTRITIONAL SUPPLEMENTS

Before taking any vitamins or nutritional supplements, talk with your doctor, who may want to test the levels of these compounds in your blood and advise you about what dose to take—or advise you not to take any at all. Be sure your physician knows what supplements you take and at what doses. The following supplements have been shown to help some women who have PMS symptoms.

• Calcium. Among nutritional supplements, calcium has the most evidence for benefit for PMS. When taken at doses of 1200 mg per day, calcium has been shown to reduce both the physical and emotional symptoms of PMS.

• Vitamin B6. Pyridoxine (vitamin B6) has possible value in ameliorating premenstrual symptoms, but it should be used with caution. Taking more than 100 mg/day of vitamin B6 can cause muscle weakness, numbness, clumsiness, and nerve damage.

• Other vitamins and supplements. Other alternative treatments that show possible benefit are *Vitex agnus-castus* (chasteberry) and St. John's wort. Many other treatments have been suggested but lack evidence of clear benefit. Vitamins D and E have proven to have some usefulness but need more research. Studies of linoleic acid (a primary ingredient in evening primrose oil) have shown mixed results in trials. There is some evidence that magnesium (200 mg/day) may reduce symptoms of fluid retention (breast tenderness, bloating, and swelling of extremities).

One word of warning about nutritional supplements like chasteberry, evening primrose oil, and St. John's wort: the FDA does not monitor the production or use of these agents, so there is potentially more risk involved in choosing to take them instead of relying on getting nutrients from food or in taking FDA-approved medications. The levels of active ingredients in nutritional supplements can vary widely between manufacturers. Many claims are made about the benefits of alternative treatments, but some of these claims are based on anecdotal evidence and may not be proven. The safety of these treatments is also not ensured. Even vitamins should be taken with caution.

EXERCISE MORE

Exercise is another lifestyle change that is widely recommended for women with PMS and PMDD. Although there has been limited research to substantiate the claim, many women with PMS say that exercise has helped them. It has been shown that aerobic exercise can increase endorphins in normal individuals. It is possible that women with PMS and PMDD who exercise show mood improvement due to an increase in endorphins. In addition, exercise can give one a sense of personal accomplishment that boosts well-being.

TRY DIFFERENT THERAPIES OR TREATMENTS

- Consider talk therapy. Psychotherapy (talk therapy) is sometimes recommended for women with PMS and PMDD. Cognitive behavioral therapy (CBT) is one approach that has been evaluated for its effectiveness for these conditions, and some evidence suggests that it may provide benefit that can be maintained. See chapters 6 and 7 for more discussion of CBT.

• Engage in relaxation and/or meditation. Relaxation training may be helpful, especially if it is combined with other approaches. Meditation is another practice that can help. Both methods address physical sensations as well as the mind and can increase one's feeling of control over what seems overwhelming. Both can be done alone or in a group, at any time, and require no equipment and minimal training.

• Try light therapy. A noninvasive treatment that has been shown to help moods is exposure to bright light (sometimes called phototherapy). This approach has been used to treat seasonal affective disorder (SAD) and may also benefit women with PMDD. Several studies have demonstrated that exposure to bright light (with a special lamp or light box) may reduce depression, irritability, and the physical symptoms of PMS/PMDD.

• Experiment with acupuncture. Acupuncture may have benefit for PMS and PMDD. In this technique, based on traditional Chinese medicine, a trained and qualified acupuncturist inserts thin needles in precisely defined sites on the body. The evidence that this treatment is effective is limited, and more study is needed.

GET EVALUATED FOR MEDICATION

Talk to your doctor about the pros and cons of various medications and dosing schedules.

• Consider the benefits of selective serotonin reuptake inhibitors. By far the most promising agents for treatment of PMDD at this time are the selective serotonin reuptake inhibitors (SSRIs). These medications have been available since the 1980s for the treatment of depression and have also been systematically studied and found consistently effective for PMDD.

- Discuss with your doctor the possibility of taking SSRIs only during the premenstrual phase. One surprising discovery about treatment of severe PMS is that SSRI medications such as Prozac (fluoxetine) are effective even when given *only* during the premenstrual phase. What makes this discovery surprising is that antidepressants take about a month to work for most patients who have depression. Many studies have confirmed the benefit of this unusual dosing approach.

- Try variable dosing. For women who have premenstrual exacerbation of depression (PMED), characterized by constant depressive symptoms that worsen premenstrually, there is also evidence that a variable dosing schedule can be beneficial. Using this approach, the dose of antidepressant is increased during the seven to ten premenstrual days. For example, if you are on 20 mg/day of Prozac, your physician may recommend that you increase your dose to 30 mg/day for the week before your period.

- Consider diuretics. Diuretics (known informally as "water pills") have been studied extensively and may have benefit for alleviating water-retention symptoms. One diuretic, Aldactone (spironolactone), failed to relieve any symptoms of PMS except bloating. Parlodel (bromocriptine) is another medication that can relieve breast tenderness, but shows little promise for the other symptoms of PMS/PMDD.

- Take a look at anxiety medications. Another option might be anxiety medications. The antianxiety agent Xanax (alprazolam) has been found to be effective for PMS in several studies when given only during the premenstrual phase. Buspar (buspirone) is another antianxiety medication that may have benefit for PMS, even when only given premenstrually. In general, anxiety medications are less effective than the SSRIs for PMS/PMDD. And, unfortunately, antianxiety agents have the potential to be addictive. They should be used with caution, preferably infrequently. Some physicians avoid prescribing them altogether for this reason.

EXPLORE HORMONAL TREATMENT OPTIONS

- Progesterone. Do not take progesterone for PMS. Progesterone is a hormone that has been prescribed as a treatment for PMS, based on the theory that it was deficient in women with this condition. However, multiple well-designed studies have failed to demonstrate any superiority of progesterone over a placebo. On the basis of these studies, progesterone should not be used as a treatment for PMS.
- Birth control pills. The thinking on birth control pills as a treatment for PMS has changed. When traditional oral contraceptives were given to women with PMS in the past, about a third seemed to improve, a third remained the same, and a third worsened. It was thought that women with premenstrual symptoms were also at high risk of developing a contraceptive-induced major depression, so some researchers and physicians advised that these agents should not be used for women with PMS. Now we know that some oral contraceptives can actually help PMS and PMDD.
- Novel contraceptives. A big change in recent years has been the introduction of novel contraceptives that have benefit for PMS. Newer combination contraceptives containing the progestin drospirenone and an estrogen may benefit women with PMS and PMDD. The FDA approved the contraceptive Yaz for PMDD in 2006 after clinical trials demonstrated that Yaz significantly reduced the symptoms of PMDD. Other contraceptives containing drospirenone may be beneficial as well but are not yet approved by the FDA: they include Ocella and Beyaz. These contraceptives increase the risk of blood clots and stroke, so they should be used with caution.

PMS SYMPTOM TRACKER   Cycle Dates: _____

Use this chart to track your PMS symptoms.

Day

Symptoms	1	2	3	4	5	6	7	8	9	10	11	12	13	14	15	16	17	18	19	20	21	22	23	24	25	26	27	28	29	30	31	32	33	34	35	36	37	38	39	40	41	42	43	44	45
period																																													
acne																																													
breast swelling and tenderness																																													
feeling tired																																													
having trouble sleeping																																													
upset stomach																																													
cramps																																													
bloating																																													
constipation																																													
diarrhea																																													
headache																																													
backache																																													
appetite changes or food cravings																																													
joint or muscle pain																																													
trouble concentrating or remembering																																													
tension, irritability, mood swings, or crying spells																																													
anxiety																																													
depression																																													
other symptoms:																																													
other symptoms:																																													
other symptoms:																																													

- Extended-cycle pills. Some extended-cycle pills may reduce the symptoms that typically occur premenstrually by reducing the number of menstrual periods. While not FDA-approved for treatment of PMS or PMDD, contraceptives such as Seasonique and Seasonale can reduce the number of menstrual periods to four a year, and Lybrel can eliminate menstrual periods entirely.

INVESTIGATE OVULATION SUPPRESSORS AND SURGERY

In women who have disabling PMDD, sometimes the recommendation is made to remove or inactivate the ovaries, which can eliminate PMDD. Essentially these interventions induce a menopausal state, which means that some women experience symptoms of menopause such as hot flashes and increased risk of osteoporosis. Suppression of ovulation may be achieved through medications or through surgical removal of the ovaries. All of the treatments that suppress ovulation carry high risks for side effects and should be reserved for severe cases of PMDD that have not responded to other treatment approaches.

- Medical options. Danocrine (danazol) is a modified progestogen that may have benefit, but side effects can be problematic. Injections of Lupron (leuprolide) have also been shown to significantly reduce premenstrual symptoms.
- Surgical options. Surgical removal of the ovaries and hysterectomy, followed by estrogen replacement, will also eliminate mood and physical symptoms associated with PMS. However, surgery is an irreversible procedure that destroys reproductive potential and, again, must be considered carefully.

•

Premenstrual disorders are real, and recognizing menstrual variations can be a significant intervention in itself. If you have

FIGURE 1. *(opposite)*   PMS SYMPTOM TRACKER   From www.womenshealth.gov, a federal government website managed by the Office on Women's Health in the Office of the Assistant Secretary for Health at the U.S. Department of Health and Human Services.

PMS or PMDD, there are treatments that can lead to significant improvement in quality of life. Start now by charting your monthly mood shifts (see figure 1). If you see a pattern of premenstrual worsening of your moods, begin using tools in this chapter such as diet and exercise. As always, consult your doctor and honestly explore your symptoms and the approaches to treatment that will work best for you.

RECOMMENDED RESOURCES

BOOKS

Diana Dell, MD, and Carol Svec. *The PMDD Phenomenon.* Columbus, Ohio: McGraw-Hill, 2003.

Diana Taylor, RN, PhD, and Stacey Colino. *Taking Back the Month: A Personalized Solution for Managing PMS and Enhancing Your Health.* New York: Perigree Trade, 2002.

WEBSITE

PMS Symptom Tracker (see figure 1):

http://www.womenshealth.gov/publications/our-publications/pms -symptom-tracker.pdf

CHAPTER 3

The Childbearing Years

Ingrid was not ready to be a mother. She was 23 years old and full of self-doubt—plus, she got little support from family or friends. She grew up in a home filled with fighting, culminating in her parents' divorce when Ingrid was ten. Her father left her mother for another woman, and her mother struggled with anger and sadness, often venting to Ingrid about her problems. As a child, Ingrid sometimes felt that she needed to take care of her mother and that she did not receive much nurturance herself.

Ingrid went to a state college and did okay. She majored in art and hoped to become an art teacher. After graduating, though, she couldn't find a teaching job and instead became a waitress. She had been living with her boyfriend for six months but had doubts about their relationship, and his occasional bad temper scared her. Her parents lived in another city and when she found out she was pregnant she was reluctant to tell them the news. Her job was low paying and she had debt from her school loans. Ingrid didn't know how she and her boyfriend could afford to take care of a child; the cost of day care would be expensive. Since she had spent little time around kids and her own childhood had been unhappy, she was scared that she would not be a good mother. Abortion was not an option for her due to her religious beliefs. She was overwhelmed thinking of all the changes in her life. She had trouble sleeping and cried easily.

Ingrid came to me for an evaluation, and I could see immediately that she was very depressed. She cried throughout the appointment and struggled to tell her story. Because she was pregnant, our treatment choices were complicated. I diagnosed her with major depression and advised her about the risks and benefits of medication during pregnancy, as well as the risks of untreated depression. I recommended therapy, and Ingrid began weekly sessions that she found very helpful. Ingrid was concerned about the risks of harming her baby through the use of an antidepressant so she chose to be treated with therapy alone until her baby was born. We planned together that she would start on an antidepressant as soon as she delivered her child. We discussed the risks and benefits of breastfeeding while on an antidepressant, and she decided that she wanted to think about it before making a decision whether to breastfeed or bottle feed her baby.

Despite her worries, Ingrid became excited as her pregnancy progressed. She grew to love the idea of being a mother and was eager to deliver. Her boyfriend was supportive, and their relationship improved.

•

From puberty until menopause, women have many choices regarding childbearing in our world today. Sexual activity may occur across a wide age range, and women have options to control when and if they have children. A variety of methods of birth control are widely available. Pregnancy may be avoided, postponed, or delayed—or, alternatively, may be difficult to achieve and the focus of much effort. Pregnancies can be terminated or may be lost. I discuss the impact of these many possible scenarios for today's women in this chapter.

Contraception

Birth control allows women to choose if and when to become pregnant. Years ago, the older generations of birth control pills were considered to be a significant risk factor for developing depression. Women who were diagnosed with or at risk for depression were advised to avoid oral contraceptives. Since then, a new generation of oral contraceptives has been developed that in some cases may instead help to prevent mood swings such as those seen in premenstrual syndromes. Most oral contraceptives include both estrogen and progestin, although there is also a progestin-only pill available for women who are unable to take estrogen. Approximately 80 percent of sexually active young women in the United States use oral contraceptives, but we have limited information on how current birth control pills affect women's moods.

A variety of contraceptive methods, such as implants and injections, alter the hormonal control of the reproductive system. An implant is a small plastic rod that releases the hormone progestin and is inserted under the skin on the arm to prevent pregnancy for up to three years. Contraceptive injections contain progestogen and last for 8 to 12 weeks. Another hormonal method of birth control is the hormonal vaginal contraceptive ring that releases estrogen and progestin for several weeks and is removed at the time of menses. Yet another option is a skin patch that releases synthetic estrogen and progestin hormones into the bloodstream and is replaced weekly. Patterns of menstrual bleeding are altered by these methods.

Another reversible method of contraception is the intrauterine device (IUD), which is a small device placed by the doctor inside the uterus to prevent pregnancy. One version of the IUD that is now in use releases a small amount of progestin each day. The IUD can stay inside the uterus for years and is highly effective.

Some women report depression as a side effect of their contraceptive, including hormonal contraceptive implants and injections. Women sometimes report stopping their birth control pills due to the apparent depression and mood changes. A subgroup of women may be more vulnerable to the mood effects of these treatments.

Barrier methods of birth control avoid the issue of mood influence, but are not as effective as hormonal methods for preventing pregnancy. These include the diaphragm or cervical cap, which are inserted prior to intercourse to cover the cervix to block sperm. Male and female condoms have the advantage of offering protection against sexually transmitted diseases. Spermicides such as foams and gels can be placed in the vagina no more than one hour prior to intercourse.

Finally, there are theoretically permanent methods of birth control that are available for those who know that they do not want to have a pregnancy in the future. These include female sterilization through tubal ligation ("tying tubes") and male sterilization through vasectomy. Both of these procedures can be done on an outpatient basis and are highly effective, although in rare instances failures can occur. The decision to undergo such an irreversible procedure is a very serious one, and should be thoughtfully considered.

Pregnancy

The confirmation of a pregnancy is dramatic news for most women. Whether the pregnancy is planned or unplanned, desired or dreaded, becoming pregnant brings physical and psychological changes. Having a child transforms your life. You begin a new stage the day you learn that you are pregnant and the focus shifts to future plans. For many, this is a joyful time ripe with promise. For others, like Ingrid, it can be an extremely difficult period.

During pregnancy, your body and mind prepare for the arrival of a baby. Anxiety about childbirth is common. You may be concerned about how to be a good mother, how to meet your expenses, and the many stresses involved with adding another family member. The pregnancy, and later the arrival of the baby, may strain your relationship with your partner. At the same time, you may receive support from others and realize that you have a new connection with many other women.

PREPARING FOR PREGNANCY

If you are hoping to become pregnant, or anticipate the possibility of pregnancy in the near future, it is wise to plan ahead. Pay attention to your nutrition. Every woman should take the vitamin folic acid (400 to 800 mcg/day, available in most multivitamins) before becoming pregnant, since folic acid reduces the possibility of certain birth defects. If you are already using a prescribed medication, talk to your doctor about the pros and cons of continuing with it if you become pregnant.

Certain medications are unsafe to use during pregnancy, and it is wise to think ahead to avoid taking them. The risk of birth defects is especially high for certain mood stabilizers (such as valproic acid and carbamazepine) as well as anxiety medications (benzodiazepines). Since many pregnancies are unplanned, it is advisable to choose a medication that has less potential for birth defects throughout the childbearing years. Specific medication risks are discussed later in this chapter.

DEPRESSION DURING PREGNANCY

Women can become depressed during pregnancy, yet recent data show that two-thirds of the time it is not diagnosed. Years ago we thought that pregnancy provided a natural protection from depression, but now we know that depression can occur. The factors that make depression more likely during pregnancy are similar to those that put women at risk at other times in their lives: genetic susceptibility, lack of support, and stress. Women who take an antidepressant and choose to stop taking it during their pregnancy are highly likely (close to 70%) to become depressed during their pregnancy.

The challenge during pregnancy is that all treatment decisions must include the potential impact on the unborn child as well as the mother. Even deciding not to treat depression with antidepressants can affect the baby. Untreated depression in the mother during pregnancy increases the risks for her baby. These risks include lower birth weights, higher risk of premature birth and birth complications, smaller head size at birth, delayed cognitive and language development, and behavioral problems.

Psychotherapy (talk therapy) is a good choice for treatment of depression during pregnancy. There is no potential for damaging side effects. A variety of short-term approaches can be effective. Therapy can help you prepare yourself for your maternal role, and your therapist can help to monitor your level of depression. For many people with mild to moderate levels of depression, therapy works as well as medication!

If therapy alone is not sufficient, the decision about whether to use medication is yours to make. There is no option that is without risks. You and your baby could potentially be affected by your untreated depression, and you and your baby could potentially be affected by exposure to medication. My suggestion is to seriously consider the risks and benefits of these options and discuss them with your partner and with your doctor. Since research is continuing on these issues, seek the latest information.

IS IT SAFE TO USE ANTIDEPRESSANT MEDICATION DURING PREGNANCY?

There is no easy answer to the question of whether to use medication to treat depression during pregnancy. Both untreated depression during pregnancy and antidepressant medications carry risks, which should be considered for each individual. It is difficult to determine the relative risks since so few studies focus on this issue. For ethical reasons, researchers cannot select some depressed pregnant women to receive a medication while other depressed women receive a placebo (random assignment to either a drug or a placebo is how drugs are tested in many other populations). Instead, we base our recommendations on the results that are observed and reported after babies have been exposed. Also, there are fewer data for new drugs, and for that reason alone they are considered more risky.

So what do we know at this time about antidepressants during pregnancy? There are several types of risk to the fetus and child from maternal antidepressants during pregnancy:

Congenital abnormalities Fortunately, this type of defect is not likely after exposure to antidepressants, but there is some risk with specific medications. The Federal Drug Administration (FDA) and the American College of Obstetricians and Gynecologists warn that use of Paxil (paroxetine) in the first trimester may be associated with increased risk of fetal birth defects and should be avoided by women who are pregnant or considering a pregnancy. In July 2015 a study conducted by the Centers for Disease Control published in *BMJ* revealed that both Paxil and Prozac (fluoxetine) taken during three months before pregnancy or the first trimester were associated with a small risk of several birth defects. In contrast, this study found no increased risks of birth defects with Celexa (citalopram), Lexapro (escitalopram), or Zoloft (sertraline).

Persistent pulmonary hypertension of the newborn (PPHN). This rare but serious defect can occur after exposure to SSRIs during late (third trimester) pregnancy. PPHN is a condition in which the blood vessels in the lungs of the newborn do not relax normally following delivery, which means that the baby does not get enough oxygen. The severity of this condition varies, but it can be dangerous and require intensive medical care and sometimes can cause death. Surviving infants may have serious consequences including delay in learning, major neurological deficits, and hearing loss. There is no known risk of PPHN from exposure to non-SSRI antidepressants or exposure to SSRIs prior to week 20 of the pregnancy.

There is controversy about the likelihood of PPHN after exposure to SSRIs. Scientific evidence has been contradictory, but a recent systematic review of the literature found that exposure to SSRIs in *late* pregnancy was associated with a slight risk of PPHN. Although PPHN has been reported twice as often in babies exposed to SSRIs during late pregnancy as in those not exposed, the absolute risk is very small (3 per 1,000 exposed infants compared with 1.2 per 1,000 rate for infants who were not exposed).

Delivery complications. There is now quite a bit of evidence that SSRI use late in pregnancy is associated with increased risks at delivery, including an increased rate of premature delivery, miscarriage, growth restriction, and low birth weight.

Post-birth poor neonatal adaptation syndrome (PNAS). PNAS refers to a cluster of abnormalities that can occur after birth: a withdrawal-like condition in the newborn including irritability, poor feeding, respiratory distress, and jitteriness. Conflicting reports exist about the likelihood of an infant developing PNAS after exposure to SSRIs. Some report that this syndrome may occur in up to 30 percent of exposed babies, and there is a consensus that the syndrome is a possible consequence of taking SSRIs. Fortunately, these symptoms are temporary and usually resolve within a couple of weeks.

Child development impairments. The most uncertain aspect of a mother taking antidepressant medication during pregnancy is the potential for long-term developmental consequences after exposure to antidepressants. Most data that have been collected so far are reassuring that language, temperament, behavior, and distractibility are not affected. This is the most difficult area to study and more data are needed.

In summary, it is important for you seek the latest information from your doctor about risks of medications taken during pregnancy.

IS IT SAFE TO USE MOOD-STABILIZING MEDICATIONS DURING PREGNANCY?

Women with bipolar disorder need to discuss medication options with their doctors prior to considering pregnancy. Some women may be able to gradually taper and discontinue their medication before conception and remain in a stable mood. However, there is an approximate 50 percent risk of relapse after stopping medication. The choices are difficult, due to the risks from the medications that are available.

Birth defects. Many mood stabilizers carry significant risk of birth defects. In particular, pregnant women and women trying to become pregnant should avoid the anticonvulsants Depakote (valproic acid) and Tegretol (carbamazepine) since they can cause neural tube defects (such as spina bifida, in which the spinal cord is not completely closed), deformities of the face and head, and difficulties with learning. If you are being treated with one of those two medications, you should discuss with your doctor the possibility of being switched to another medication before you try to become pregnant in order to reduce the risk of harm to your baby.

Lamictal (lamotrigine) is another mood stabilizer that is sometimes used for bipolar disorder. Exposure to this medication during pregnancy slightly increases the risk of cleft lip or cleft palate (total risk about 8.9 per 1,000, or .89%).

Cardiac defects. Eskalith (lithium) is another mood stabilizer that is often used to treat bipolar disorder. Lithium is considered safer than the anticonvulsants discussed in the previous paragraph, but it has a small risk (0.05 to 0.1%) of causing a cardiac defect if given during the first trimester of pregnancy. This risk should be carefully weighed against the possibility of relapse, since becoming more ill can also create danger for both the mother and baby.

For further discussion of mood-stabilizing medications, see chapter 9 on bipolar disorder.

Postpartum Depression

Sofia was upbeat and cheerful before she had her baby. She had never been depressed and didn't really understand people "like that." She was energetic and enjoyed being active with her husband and friends.

Sofia woke up on the fourth day after she gave birth with a gnawing sense of dread. It was a dramatic change; more than a bad day. The feeling persisted. She became severely anxious and worried constantly. She cried easily, for entire days if she let herself, and it became harder and harder to resist crying. She lost her sense of hope for the future. She no longer felt excited about anything.

It took Sofia a long time to find and respond to the right help. Before she came to me, she talked to her obstetrician-gynecologist about her feelings and felt that he was dismissive. He told her to avoid sugar and said that her feelings would just go away in time. She saw a psychiatrist but did not respond to the treatment. She started searching on the Internet for support and for treatment ideas.

I evaluated Sofia when she was already several months postpartum, and I was struck by the severity of her depression and anxiety. Her appointments were lengthy because she brought long lists of concerns and questions. The first antidepressant we chose did not work well for her. Eventually we found the combination of psychotherapy and fluoxetine (Prozac) helped a lot.

Sofia fully recovered and regained her energy. She and her husband decided that they wanted a second child. We discussed the risks of another episode of depression as well as the risks of treatment with her antidepressant during pregnancy. Sofia chose to get off her medication before becoming pregnant, and did okay during the pregnancy. At the second postpartum day, she felt the awful feelings of depression coming back, but since we had restarted the fluoxetine, her depression resolved quickly. She was able to avoid a full episode of postpartum depression after her second child was born.

The experience of depression changed Sofia's life. She blames the depression in part for how her marriage unraveled; she wound up divorcing a few years later. She wonders if her daughter was harmed by the depression during her first year. On the positive side, she has gained understanding and compassion for others who suffer from depression and other emotional problems. She has become an advocate for educating others with depression. She is now happy, remarried, and doing well.

WHAT HAPPENS POSTPARTUM?

Sofia was surprised to find herself depressed after the birth of her child, at a time that was supposed to be joyful. This is the case for many women who develop postpartum depression. It is the first time many women experience depression, and they don't understand what is happening to them. For women who have been depressed in the past, the return of depression at this time is confusing. Most women feel guilty about having such feelings, as well as ashamed. The baby shower was only weeks ago and everyone was so happy. How can they make sense of the bad feelings?

The risk for depression increases after childbirth, especially for women with a history of depression. It is widely believed that the dramatic shifts in hormone levels that occur at the time of delivery interact with an underlying vulnerability in some women to trigger depression. Relationship problems, financial issues, and other stressors can increase the risk as well.

Postpartum depression is very different from the common but temporary phenomenon nicknamed "baby blues." As many as 50 to 70 percent of women have a brief period of moodiness after giving birth that resolves spontaneously after a few days. They may feel more sensitive and cry easily at this time, but do not have all the other symptoms of major depression.

In contrast, the 10 to 15 percent of women who develop postpartum depression have the symptoms of major depression (see chapter 6 for a full discussion of major depression). What primarily sets these women apart from other people with depression is that their depression began after delivery. Many new mothers who have major depression also have high levels of anxiety and obsessions.

Awareness of the possibility of postpartum depression has improved in recent years, in large part due to the courage of individuals such as Brooke Shields, who publicly shared her experience. Knowing that postpartum depression has affected other women, and understanding that it is a risk, can help women and their families recognize when it happens to them as well.

Women who have a family history of postpartum depression, or who have a personal history of depression, should watch their mood closely after childbirth. Common symptoms of postpartum depression are changes in sleep and appetite, difficulty concentrating, fatigue, loss of interests, and inability to feel pleasure. Sometimes suicidal thoughts can occur. Identifying and treating the illness early does much to diminish its harm.

A small percentage of women (1 or 2 out of 1,000) develop postpartum psychosis after delivery. In this illness, women may hear voices or see things that are not there. They may become paranoid and believe that others are trying to hurt them. They may develop delusions, which are false beliefs. Sometimes they have thoughts about harming the baby. Tragic stories about postpartum women killing their children have led the public to fear this disorder. Postpartum psychosis is considered a psychiatric emergency and often requires hospitalization to protect the safety of both the mother and her children.

IS IT SAFE TO USE ANTIDEPRESSANTS WHILE BREASTFEEDING?

What should a woman do about breastfeeding if she is prescribed and needs to take an antidepressant? This is an important decision for women with postpartum depression. This question is complex, and without easy answers.

Breast milk has many benefits for the health of the baby and for the bonding between mother and child. It transfers the mother's immunity to the baby and is nature's way for mothers to give their children protection against disease. Mother-baby bonding through breastfeeding has been shown to give important psychological benefits to the child.

There is evidence that antidepressants taken while nursing get transmitted into breast milk, but the quantities of this medication are miniscule. There is no clear evidence that this small amount of exposure results in damage to the baby.

Ultimately, this is another situation in which the mother and her partner need to consult with the woman's psychiatrist and infant's pediatrician, weigh the risks of infant exposure to medications (which are not clearly known) versus the benefits of nursing, and make their own choices. Some new mothers who are prescribed antidepressants prefer to "play it safe" and choose bottle feeding to avoid any potential impact of medication. Others decide that the nursing benefits for the physical and emotional health of the baby outweigh possible risks that have not been proved.

Miscarriage

Miscarriage is an emotionally painful experience. The woman who has become pregnant and is progressing through the stages of her pregnancy may be full of anticipation and hope about her future child. If she has begun to wear her maternity clothes, she likely has many conversations with others about what is happening. Her focus starts to shift toward this new person who is growing in her uterus, and she starts to prepare herself emotionally and physically for the arrival. She may start to create a nursery for the baby, and to buy clothing and supplies. Friends and family may give her a baby shower. If she has other children, she will see their reactions to her changing appearance and to the idea of a new sibling. She and her husband or partner will have evolving feelings about the pregnancy as they adjust their expectations for family life.

Losing your baby to miscarriage in the midst of the emotions of pregnancy can be devastating. Miscarriage often happens unexpectedly and can be frightening and painful, with a huge sense of loss. It is common for miscarriages to elicit feelings of guilt in the mother. You are likely to rethink your actions and to blame yourself for the loss, whether these thoughts are rational or not. You may develop superstitious thinking about why you lost the baby. You may or may not feel supported by your husband and family. Others may share in your grief and may not know how to manage their own feelings. After a miscarriage, friends and family may make comments that are meant to be helpful but instead are experienced as hurtful.

If this was a first pregnancy, the role of new mother is suddenly removed. You may not want to explain to others what happened to you. What was recently a joyous time can quickly become a sad one.

In addition to the fact that this is a loss that needs to be grieved, miscarriage is associated with changes in hormone levels that are similar to the changes that occur with full-term pregnancy. These hormonal changes may trigger depression in some women. In short, there are several reasons to be on the watch for the development of depression after a miscarriage.

Abortion

Choosing to have an abortion is an intensely personal decision with long-term consequences. We live in an era when abortion is legal but highly controversial. Political campaigns frequently emphasize the opinions of the candidate on whether laws about abortion should be retained or changed. Moral judgments are everywhere. Women who seek abortions and doctors who provide this procedure are attacked as "murderers" and may be physically threatened. Passions run high around this topic.

A woman who decides to seek an abortion is often confronted with doubts and harsh realities. She may not feel capable of providing a baby with the nurturance needed at this point in her own life. She may lack financial and emotional support. She may be frightened by the responsibility. She may think that her future career options will be limited by having a baby, or that she will not be able to cope with the additional stress. She may never have experienced good role modeling for mothering and family life and may fear what her life will become if she is a mother. She may feel pressured by the baby's father to terminate the pregnancy. She may feel that she has no options. She may be confused and concerned about making "the right choice."

The ready availability of abortion allows women to make this decision fairly independently. Some women regret their choice to abort for many years. They may experience feelings of guilt and shame. It may become a secret that they carry. Other women are able to move on with their lives and are grateful that they had the option to postpone motherhood at a time when they did not feel ready. There is debate within the field of women's mental health about the psychological consequences of abortion, and women's reactions vary greatly.

Infertility

Infertility can cause emotional anguish and be associated with depression. This common problem affects about 10 percent of women in the childbearing years. Infertility is often associated with feelings of inadequacy, and may cause conflict within the couple. They may feel guilt, and blame each other and themselves for not being able to get pregnant. Couples may spend substantial time, money, and effort trying to conceive. An infertile mother or couple may find it difficult to be around pregnant women and new parents. They can feel isolated and may have difficulty coping with events that highlight parenting, such as baby showers and Mother's and Father's Day celebrations.

The first step to address this problem is to have a fertility specialist determine the cause. Infertility may be due to the woman, the man, or the couple. Treatment options for women include oral medication or hormone injections to stimulate the ovaries to release eggs, artificial insemination, surgery for blocked or damaged fallopian tubes, and laparoscopic surgery to remove uterine tissue that has grown in the abdomen. Treatment for problems associated with the man includes collecting and concentrating sperm and then introducing it through artificial insemination.

If these methods do not work or are not chosen, the couple may opt for in vitro fertilization (IVF), in which eggs are fertilized outside the woman's body and then placed into the woman's uterus, through the cervix. Another method is sperm injection, in which one sperm is injected into one egg outside the woman's body. If fertilization occurs, the doctor places the embryo in the woman's uterus.

If couples do not achieve pregnancy from infertility treatments, they may choose to use a third party to donate the egg and/or the sperm. If the woman is unable to carry a pregnancy to term and has not been able to produce healthy eggs, she may seek a surrogate who can be inseminated with sperm from the male partner. Another option is for an embryo to be implanted into another woman (called a gestational carrier) if the infertile woman produces healthy eggs but has been unable to carry a pregnancy to term.

Infertility treatments are expensive and often not covered by insurance. Having to make a choice among the variety of fertility treatments may feel overwhelming.

Infertility and depression are intimately related. There is evidence that women are less likely to conceive when they are depressed or stressed. As you would expect, women who have problems with fertility are likely to worry and be sad. They also may have conflict within their relationship due to this stress. Both partners may have feelings of inadequacy, sadness, anger, embarrassment, and frustration. If hormones are prescribed for the woman in fertility treatment, they may cause her to be more moody. Infertility may be one of the stresses that lead a woman to develop depression. Treatment of the depression may improve the likelihood of conception. Women who struggle with infertility should pay attention to their emotions as well as their bodies and seek help as needed.

Newer methods of assisted reproduction can be applied in other situations as well. Women undergoing chemotherapy and/or radiation treatment may choose to preserve their eggs and their ovarian tissue through freezing until a later date; couples using IVF may create embryos that are saved for the future; gay couples may use IVF or surrogates to have their own biological children. In 2014, the first baby was born after a successful uterine transplant to a woman born with functioning ovaries but no uterus. The world is changing and there are many technological advances that can affect women during the childbearing years.

Adoption

Some women pursue adoption as the first route to motherhood. For others, it is the last resort. No matter how the decision is made, the psychological issues associated with adoption are many.

For those who actively choose adoption, the reason may be a concern about overpopulation or a desire to give a better life to a child who is orphaned or whose parents are unable to care for him or her. For gay couples who choose not to use assisted reproductive technologies it offers another option to family building.

For some who have struggled with making a family—for example, infertile couples—it may be the only path left. They may progress from their grief about their own infertility into the joy of finding a child who needs parents. The process may be lengthy and anxiety-producing, since there are often delays, legal paperwork, and the lurking fear that the biological parents might appear and want to reclaim their child. Women who have been unable to give birth may have a lingering sadness until they are fully able to accept and embrace the idea of adoption and their new family member.

Pregnant women may elect to place their baby for adoption if they feel unable to adequately parent their child. Mothers who make this choice may feel guilty about the decision for many years or a lifetime. They may also feel shame and hide this choice from others in fear of being judged. Alternatively, some who relinquish their babies recognize that this was the best option for the children as well as for themselves.

Adoptive parents vary in their degree of openness with their children about the adoption. Many parents tell their children from an early age that they were adopted, and add that they were specially chosen and very much desired. Regardless of how the adoptive parents communicate with their child, most children eventually question their origins and are curious about their biological parents. Adolescents as well as adults may seek out their birth parents to give themselves a greater understanding of their background.

Reactions of biological parents to communications with their child who was placed for adoption vary greatly and can have a significant impact on the child. Some parents are reluctant to acknowledge the child they relinquished, especially if the pregnancy was a secret at the time and current family members are unaware of it. Other parents are open to accepting and embracing the child they gave birth to years ago. Sometimes it is the biological parent who seeks out the child years later and asks for communication or for a meeting. Our society has become much more open about adoption, and there are many possible relationships that can develop.

Many adopted children are grateful to their adoptive parents for choosing to raise them. They may develop an appreciation of the sacrifice made by the biological mother as well. On the other hand, adopted children may harbor anger and resentment toward their biological parents. They may feel rejected and abandoned, and these feelings may affect their self-esteem for many years. These feelings may be especially strong if they were removed from their biological parents because of abuse or neglect. If they were placed into the foster care system, they may have experienced instability or trauma. It is not unusual for children who were adopted to have a mixture of feelings about their background.

Adopted children may have more risk for developing depression if they inherited that vulnerability from their biological parents, and also if they were raised by an adoptive mother who is herself depressed. In addition, psychological reactions to the concept of adoption may contribute to depression in the child. The child may feel that she was rejected due to some defect in herself, or may feel hurt by the belief that her biological mother did not love her enough to keep her. Adoptive parents can help to overcome such depressive thoughts in the child by reassuring her of how much they wanted her, chose her, and love her.

•

WHAT CAN YOU DO TO PREVENT AND TREAT DEPRESSION IN THE CHILDBEARING YEARS?

- Seek sources of support *before* delivering your baby. Anticipate that your level of stress will increase and plan ahead for taking breaks from your responsibilities and finding time for yourself.

- If you become depressed during pregnancy, consider the various forms of treatment for depression discussed in chapter 6. Psychotherapy can be especially helpful at this stage since your life priorities have transformed overnight and you may need some help in thinking through your changes. Relaxation and meditation may help restore your sense of balance. Antidepressants can be helpful as well. The combination of medication and therapy may be the best choice for many women. Discuss safety issues about the choice of medication with your obstetrician.
- Be alert for symptoms of depression that occur after childbirth, especially if you have ever been depressed before.
- If you have a past history of postpartum depression, talk to your doctor about starting on an antidepressant soon after delivery.

The busy childbearing years can be some of the most challenging. You may feel pulled in many directions and may neglect your own needs. Finding ways to nurture yourself is important for maintaining your equilibrium during this time of your life. Experiences related to childbearing and the stresses of parenting can be overwhelming at times. These are also years when your own identity is evolving. You progress from the uncertain identity of the adolescent, into the relative freedom and independence of young adulthood, and often into the new responsibilities of parenthood. Throughout these stages, be alert for possible symptoms of anxiety and depression as discussed in chapters 6 and 7. Everyone experiences stress, but with proactive efforts you can take care of yourself and preserve your emotional balance.

RECOMMENDED RESOURCES

BOOKS

Shoshana Bennett, PhD, and Pec Indman, EdD, MFT. *Beyond the Blues: A Guide to Understanding and Treating Prenatal and Postpartum Depression.* San Jose, CA: Moodswings Press, 2003.

Kevin Gyoerkoe, PsyD, and Pamela Wiegartz, PhD. *The Pregnancy and Postpartum Anxiety Workbook: Practical Skills to Help You Overcome Anxiety, Worry, Panic Attacks, Obsessions and Compulsions.* Oakland, CA: New Harbinger Publications, 2009.

Shaila Misri, MD. *Pregnancy Blues: What Every Woman Needs to Know About Depression During Pregnancy.* New York: Delacorte Press, 2005.

Ruta Nonacs, MD, PhD. *A Deeper Shade of Blue: A Woman's Guide to Recognizing and Treating Depression in Her Childbearing Years.* New York: Simon and Schuster, 2006.

WEBSITES

For Postpartum Support International: www.postpartum.net

For grief following miscarriage and other early child loss: www.silentgrief.com

For further information on contraception, pregnancy, postpartum conditions, or infertility, see the patient page of the American College of Obstetricians and Gynecologists website: www.acog.org/Patients

- About medication safety during pregnancy

    OTIS (Organization of Teratology Information Specialists): www.otispregnancy.org

    Motherisk: www.motherisk.org

CHAPTER 4

The Menopausal Transition and Beyond

Anna was approaching fifty when she became my patient. She told me she was feeling unfulfilled, anxious, and depressed. She felt unappreciated by her husband of 20 years. They no longer had fun together and hadn't had sex for over a year. She felt guilty about her mother, who was unhappy in her nursing home. She feared the "empty nest" which was looming—her youngest child would be leaving for college in another year. She felt the need for a new direction.

Anna had a relatively happy childhood. She had graduated from college and worked for several years as an office manager before having children. Anna had been a homemaker for years now, but wondered what she would do with herself when her youngest son left for college. In the last few years, her son had been pulling away from her and she was feeling lonelier. Her husband was busy with his job. She had started to doubt her worth.

When I first suggested therapy, Anna was reluctant since she felt that she was "just complaining" and didn't deserve help. She wondered if her unhappiness was due to menopause, since her menstrual periods had become irregular. She had a few friends but did not see them often and was reluctant to confide in them what she was going through.

Anna has been in therapy for some time and finds it helpful. She realized that she was putting everyone else's needs above her own and has started to pursue old interests again. She signed up for a photography course and is considering trying to find work as a photographer. She has made time with friends a priority. She talked to her husband about her feelings, and they are becoming closer.

The Sandwich Generation

Women who are Anna's age and in this stage of life face multiple challenges. Many of them are caught in the middle between their parents' and their children's needs. These are the women who constitute the "sandwich generation." They may have time-consuming and draining caregiving responsibilities.

If they work outside the home, that's another set of demands. They may feel stuck at a job where they are not appreciated and unlikely to be promoted. If they are coupled, there are often relationship issues to deal with. They or their partner may have new health issues. If they are currently without a partner, they question whether they will ever find another meaningful relationship. They may be fearful of growing old alone. Feeling isolated and feeling stuck in our circumstances, and unsure of how to find support from others, makes us feel sad and stressed.

Caring for elderly parents can be especially challenging. Resources may be limited and information difficult to come by. Over time, our parents' health problems are likely to worsen. Many elderly people experience cognitive decline; some develop Alzheimer's disease or other dementia. They may become irritable and demanding, frustrated with their loss of autonomy and inability to participate in activities like they used to. Midlife women often are handed, and often take, responsibility for finding solutions for their parents' evolving needs. This responsibility can include responding to medical emergencies, persuading parents when a change in living arrangement is needed, and helping parents to accept a loss of independence. The aging process often includes a return to a more childlike stage of dependence, and the midlife woman may find herself essentially parenting her own parents. The elderly parent may or may not welcome her help.

For the sandwich generation woman, caring for her aging parents may feel like a burden on top of the need to care for her own children and sometimes even grandchildren. Women who are raising children alone, or whose partners are unable or unwilling to help in these multiple roles, have even more demands. Many women in their fifties and sixties find themselves looking after the oldest and youngest members of their extended family, just at the time when they may be starting to think about their own retirement.

Increasing numbers of grandparents now head households that include their grandchildren. In 1995, according to the U.S. Census Bureau, 4 million children lived in a household headed by a grandparent, which was a 40 percent increase over the previous decade. By 2010, data indicated a further increase, to 4.9 million children under age 18 living in grandparent-headed households. Many factors may explain the growing trend toward shared multigenerational homes. Economic pressures, shortages in the housing market, and lack of employment opportunities give many families few options. High divorce rates also contribute to the number of families who seek help from older—and younger—generations.

These expanded responsibilities for the midlife woman create financial, health, housing, educational, and work dilemmas. She is the problem solver for family members of various ages. She may be faced with attending PTA meetings for her grandchild, taking her mother to the emergency room, looking for a nursing home for her father, and cooking meals for everyone while juggling her own work responsibilities. Taking care of her own physical health, much less her emotional health, is often the lowest priority.

The multigenerational family certainly can have its rewards. Midlife women in this sandwich generation situation may develop a deep appreciation for the additional time they have been given with family members. Closeness develops with time together, yet these women find themselves with job descriptions much larger than they expected for this stage of their lives. Because they may have difficulty envisioning any relief, these women are under tremendous stress and at greater risk for depression as well as anxiety.

The Empty Nest

Women at midlife may find themselves left alone after years of caring for others and raising a family. Many younger women live in fear of the "empty nest." When children are able to successfully "launch," the midlife woman faces a major life change. Some mothers mourn the loss of the daily presence of their child. They may long for earlier days when their son or daughter was closer and more a part of their everyday routine. They may feel that they are no longer needed and have anxiety about how they will handle this change. The departure of children can lead to perceiving a loss of identity and meaning. For women who are divorced or widowed the home may seem especially empty, and they may feel alone. Fortunately for most women, adapting to the empty nest is easier than they anticipated.

In the absence of children the spotlight shifts onto the marriage of the parents. Sometimes parents realize that they have grown apart over time while they were focusing their energy on their children. There are many examples of midlife spouses who decide to leave their marriage for someone else. Women may also decide at the time of midlife that the dissatisfactions that they have had with their marriage over the years are no longer acceptable or tolerable. They may have waited until their children were out of the house to make a decision and take action. Divorces at midlife are common. For many women, the midlife years are a difficult challenge. They may feel less attractive and more isolated. They may become depressed and anxious. Some begin to drink more, to cope with their emotions.

In other cases, the launching of children frees the parents to rediscover themselves as individuals and as a couple. Some feel relief that they have fulfilled their parental responsibilities and appreciate the freedom to pursue their own interests. For some couples, the empty nest can be very enjoyable.

Ideally by midlife women have developed more confidence in themselves and are less concerned by the opinions of others. If they do find themselves alone, they may be able to embrace their freedom and develop their own interests. They may socialize more, develop new hobbies, and travel. Some pursue different careers or continue their education. They may start volunteering or become more actively involved with their church, temple, or other religious organization. Women's friendships with other women are an important component of their lives throughout the life cycle. Empty nesters may have an even stronger need for the support of their women friends. Health problems, family concerns, marital changes, and work issues are pressing for women at this age, and relationships continue to be a valuable key to mental health.

Changes in Your Body

One midlife stress is that the changes in a woman's body make it hard for her to ignore the aging process. Her physical abilities start to decline. Wrinkles appear. Breasts sag. Joints may start to ache. Hair turns gray. Vision worsens and she may need to wear glasses for the first time in her life (at least for reading). New medical issues may include high blood pressure or diabetes.

Body image is a problem for many women throughout the life cycle. As women reach midlife, many mourn the loss of their younger appearance. Women also are faced with the reality that others may find them less attractive. Some, seeking to reverse the aging process, may turn to cosmetic surgery or Botox injections. Other women are more accepting of the changes in their body.

Weight gain is also common at midlife and is associated with other health issues. By midlife, it is not unusual for women to weigh significantly more than they did in their twenties. One-third of Americans are obese. There is a correlation between obesity and numerous health problems, including diabetes, coronary artery disease, strokes, obstructive sleep apnea, hypertension, chronic kidney disease, gout, osteoarthritis, and gallbladder disease. In addition, a number of cancers have been linked to obesity, including endometrial, breast, kidney, esophageal, gallbladder, and colon cancers.

Women at midlife have the opportunity to improve their health by joining others in the trend toward better health and fitness in our society. Those who are able to follow an exercise routine are much more likely to feel confident in their bodies and to have improved moods.

Sexuality is another area of change for the midlife woman. With menopause, she no longer has to be concerned about contraception or becoming pregnant. This can be very freeing. On the other hand, she is likely to develop symptoms such as vaginal dryness that make sexual functioning more difficult. Some women at this stage experience a decline in their interest in sexuality, but others enjoy this aspect of their lives even more.

Perimenopause and Menopause

The hormonal changes that occur at this time of life are another piece of the puzzle that may be hard to understand. Menopause is defined as the time in a woman's life when menstruation permanently stops. The age at which menopause occurs varies, but typically ranges from age 47 to age 55. During the seven to ten years before the cessation of menstruation, a woman is said to be in perimenopause. During this time, her ovaries decline in their functioning. This decline is irregular, may vary from month to month, and has an impact on her moods.

Years ago it was thought that women were more at risk for depression when they reached menopause, and this phenomenon was called "involutional melancholia." More recent evidence indicates that it is not the time of menopause that is associated with increased risk of depression, but instead the seven to ten years before menopause—again, that perimenopause period. Menopause itself may instead be a time of relief—the term "postmenopausal zest" was coined by Margaret Mead to describe this phase. Women are more at risk for depression during perimenopause, and this is especially true for women who have a past history of major depression. In addition, women who have a past history of PMS or postpartum depression are more at risk for depression during the menopausal transition. PMS may also worsen during perimenopause before menstruation ceases. A woman's physical and mental health are vulnerable at this stage.

The decline in levels of estrogen, as the ovaries decrease their function, results in a number of symptoms. Hot flashes, night sweats, insomnia, physical aches, and fatigue are common during the menopausal transition. Headaches and backaches, shortness of breath, breast tenderness, weight gain, thinning of the skin and hair, dizziness, heart palpitations, and muscle and joint pain may occur. Vaginal atrophy may cause itching, burning, discharge, and painful intercourse for some women. Urinary incontinence and frequent urination can be problems. Bones may become weaker and develop osteoporosis. Emotional symptoms women experience during perimenopause and menopause include irritability, anxiety, decreased motivation, insomnia, and depressed mood. All of these symptoms may be caused by the declining presence of estrogen, which in turn affects brain levels of serotonin.

Hormone Replacement Treatments

Hormone replacement therapy (HRT) has become controversial in the last decade. The unexpected results of a poorly designed study caused many women and doctors to fear using these medications that can relieve the symptoms of menopause.

Decisions about whether to use HRT and which specific HRT medication to choose are complex. HRT medications affect many organ systems. There are multiple risks and benefits to be considered, and recommendations will evolve as more research is done.

HRT includes various combinations of both estrogen and progesterone. Progesterone reduces the risk of inducing cancer of the endometrium (lining of the uterus). Women who have had a hysterectomy do not need the progesterone component since they no longer have a uterus.

Initially, HRT was thought to protect against heart disease and osteoporosis, and it was widely recommended. For women with an intact uterus, combination HRT was recommended, that included estrogen and progesterone. Women who had had a hysterectomy were often treated with estrogen alone. That recommendation changed after an unexpected study finding from a research project known as the Women's Health Initiative (WHI).

The WHI was a large multicenter trial examining the benefits and risks from combined estrogen plus progestin HRT for heart disease, stroke, and breast cancer. This study was abruptly discontinued in May 2002 when preliminary results suggested that women receiving HRT were demonstrating more instead of less risk for heart attack and stroke. Invasive breast cancer and pulmonary embolisms were also more common in the women on HRT.

News of this prematurely discontinued study spread like wildfire. Talk shows and news stories extended warnings to menopausal women that the HRT pills they were taking might be increasing instead of decreasing their risk of heart disease and stroke. Many women were alarmed by this news and stopped their HRT soon thereafter. For a time, HRT was widely condemned as dangerous for women at menopause and was no longer recommended for prevention of chronic diseases. For women with menopausal symptoms such as hot flashes and vaginal dryness, professional organizations recommended using a dose as low as possible for as short a duration as possible.

Research on HRT was also affected by the WHI trial. HRT quickly became seen as a dangerous and risky treatment for women during the menopausal transition, and research on this topic was stalled. The WHI has been criticized for its study design and especially for the fact that its results were over-interpreted. The women in the WHI study were older and postmenopausal, with an average age of 63, and therefore not a good group in which to evaluate the effectiveness and safety of HRT for younger women approaching menopause.

These recommendations changed again in mid-2007 when WHI investigators reevaluated the risks and benefits from HRT. Age was identified as a major factor in this analysis, and only breast cancer risk remained as a contraindication for HRT. Because of the very low rate of cardiovascular events and stroke prior to age 60, HRT at the age of menopause is no longer seen as unsafe. Currently HRT is recommended to ease menopausal symptoms, but still only for the shortest time, due to long-term risks for heart attacks, strokes, blood clots, and breast cancer.

Needless to say, the controversies about HRT have generated considerable confusion and debate among doctors and among women about what is their best option at the age of menopause. It is to be hoped more research in years to come will shed further light on this controversy.

SSRI medications that are used for depression may also treat menopausal symptoms such as hot flashes. In 2013 the FDA approved the release of Brisdelle, which is a new brand name for the antidepressant paroxetine (Paxil). Other SSRIs and the antidepressant venlafaxine (Effexor) can relieve hot flashes as well and are attractive alternatives for women who are afraid of taking HRT after the controversies that have developed or for a health reason such as a genetic predisposition to breast cancer.

How Does Hormone Replacement Therapy Affect the Mood?

Studies have shown that the estrogen component of HRT is protective of the mood. Estrogen has been called "nature's psychoprotectant." Progesterone, in contrast, decreases the benefit from estrogen on the mood in a dose-dependent fashion. In other words, the more progesterone that is taken together with the estrogen in HRT, the less benefit HRT will have for the mood. For women who are taking an antidepressant for depression, effectiveness can be increased with the addition of HRT that includes estrogen.

If you are considering whether to take HRT, or if you are already taking HRT but also have depression, it may be helpful for you to discuss with your doctor any problems you have had with your mood. The relative proportion of estrogen to progesterone in different hormone replacement therapies can vary greatly. For women with mood problems, it may be helpful to seek a larger proportion of estrogen.

Seeking Help at Midlife

Midlife is a time when women may need help. Problems with depression, anxiety, and substance abuse may overwhelm them. All of the changes in life circumstance that have been discussed in this chapter may result in mood changes that may benefit from treatment. Chapters 6, 7, and 8 discuss the problems of depression, anxiety, and substance abuse in more depth. Help is available, and women can regain their balance when needed. You are not alone in the struggle.

Midlife Reflections and Potential Joy

Midlife brings with it the increased recognition that life is finite. Friends and acquaintances our same age pass away. We think more about our values and the meaning of life. Vanity, status, and material possessions may diminish in importance for women in midlife. Some women undergo a spiritual awakening. The flip side of experiencing loss is an increased appreciation of all that is life.

So far I have emphasized the risks for depression and anxiety. Even so, there is evidence that many women who are at midlife experience an increase in their level of confidence and a sense of hopefulness about the future. With our general extended lifespan, we may have many more years of living than previous generations of women, and many women are seizing opportunities in this additional season of life.

As women in midlife establish a greater sense of their own abilities and independence, they may embrace this stage of life. No longer do they need to worry about the possibility of pregnancy or about monthly mood swings due to PMS. As their children become launched, they are free to explore other interests. They may feel at liberty to expand the "masculine" sides of themselves, to be less concerned with pleasing others and better able to make their own choices. They may regain the sense of adventure and athleticism that they had enjoyed earlier in life. With the right attitude (and some luck), the midlife years can be a time when we become our true selves and pursue our own dreams.

•

In summary, the menopausal transition can be physically and emotionally challenging. As a member of the "sandwich generation" you may find yourself caring for elderly parents and young children simultaneously. As children grow up and leave the home, transitions take place, and again your identity evolves. The process of aging eventually is evident to all of us, with changes in appearance and health that we must accept. Life has a way of giving us stresses and losses, and over the years we need to learn to adapt to them in order to survive. We can lose our balance by becoming overly isolated on the one hand, or by becoming depleted and drained by competing demands. Maintaining our balance requires that we allow ourselves to set limits and seek support as needed, and that we take care of ourselves both physically and emotionally.

RECOMMENDED RESOURCES

BOOKS
Jean Shinoda Bolen, MD. *Crones Don't Whine: Concentrated Wisdom for Juicy Women.* York Beach, ME: Conari Press, 2003.
Julia Schlam Edelman, MD, FACOG. *Menopause Matters: Your Guide to a Long and Healthy Life.* Baltimore: Johns Hopkins University Press, 2010.
Jane Fonda. *Prime Time: Love, Health, Sex, Fitness, Friendship, Spirit, Making the Most of All of Your Life.* New York: Random House, 2011.

Gail Sheehy. *New Passages: Mapping Your Life across Time.* New York: Random House, 2011.

Kathryn Simpson, MS, and Dale Bredesen, MD. *The Perimenopause and Menopause Workbook: A Comprehensive, Personalized Guide to Hormone Health.* Oakland, CA: New Harbinger Publications, 2006.

CHAPTER 5

The Senior Years

Mia just turned 85, and her family celebrated with a birthday party at her assisted living facility. She was so glad to be able to see her children doing well and to be a part of the lives of her grandchildren.

Mia knows that she has lived a full life. She and her husband, Ben, enjoyed their family, their friends, and each other. They both retired in their sixties and drove a recreational vehicle around the country visiting state and national parks, stopping with friends along the way. Then Ben became ill with cancer, and Mia cared for him until his death several years later.

Now Mia is struggling. Although it's been many years since Ben died, she misses her husband. She has made friends with a couple of neighbors down the hall and her family visits weekly, but much of the time she feels very lonely. She fears that she is a burden to her family and tries not to ask for much. Her knees hurt, she has little energy, she has heart disease, and she sleeps poorly. She cries occasionally. She tells herself that she would rather be dead than to be a worry to her family. She tries not to complain, but she is sad that they do not visit more often.

Issues in Late Life

Mia's generation faces many challenges. We live in a society that does not revere the elderly, as many other cultures do. Often families become geographically separated, so children and grandchildren may not live near each other or their parents as was common years ago. Even when families are in the same town, it is less likely nowadays that the elderly family members will live in the same household with other family. Losses—family members and friends—accumulate over time, and someone who lives to old age is likely to have endured a number of losses.

The longer you live, the more likely you are to have health issues. Some of these issues may be life threatening, such as cancer and heart disease. You may have to undergo chemotherapy, radiation treatment, or surgeries. Other health problems are more chronic and must be endured over years. You may have aches and pains that make it harder to climb stairs or take a walk. You likely have less energy and can't accomplish as much in a day as you did when you were younger. You may find it harder to catch your breath. Balance problems and muscle weakness make you vulnerable to falls.

Many older women become isolated. If you live alone, you may crave contact with others. Or you may be comfortable living on your own and not realize that you have become so detached. You may resist the thought of reaching out to others, fearing they will not want to spend time with you. Your senses are likely to be in decline. You may have more difficulty hearing, which increases your sense of isolation. You may have worsening vision, especially at night. In many ways it may seem easier to stay home.

Many elderly people live in settings where others surround them, yet they may still feel lonely. Retirement communities, independent and assisted living facilities, and nursing homes have become common residential arrangements in the senior years. Since women live longer than men, the population of these communities is predominantly female. Women may find kindred spirits in such settings, and if they are lucky may find friendships. Others feel extremely alone.

Unresolved issues from earlier in life may continue to affect you. You may feel angry or sad about relationships, such as with your romantic partners or children. You may have feelings about your childhood that continue to influence you, especially if you experienced trauma or abuse. Even though decades have passed, the pain from childhood may still have an impact.

Loss occurs on many levels over time. In addition to losing loved ones who have died, you may have lost your home and your previous roles in life. Changes in your appearance may feel like a loss. You may gradually shift into a more dependent relationship with your own children, so that they become your caregivers. This is a big contrast from earlier years, when you cared for them.

The transition into old age can be hard to accept, especially if you are a woman who has previously prided yourself on tending to the needs of others. Caring for others is a major component of your sense of self. You may take great pleasure and pride in making the meals and nurturing the family. You may be resistant to having others help you with daily tasks. Allowing someone else to take care of you may not be what you want at all.

You may be especially reluctant to quit driving. This is a thorny issue for families. Driving is a convenience, and for most people it also represents freedom and independence. Family members are likely to be the first to recognize that your driving skills are declining. They worry for your safety. They have concerns about the safety of others and liability if you have an accident. At the same time, family may dread the thought of confronting you with this issue and also of becoming the ones who must provide your transportation to doctors' appointments, shopping, religious services, and social outings.

Mental functioning starts to mildly or significantly decline in the senior years. Most women will be more forgetful and slower to react. For some women, old age may be accompanied by significant memory loss and confusion. If dementia does start to develop, it may progress gradually or quickly. You may be reluctant to admit that you are having difficulty and may try to hide it from others. Alternatively, you may worry that you are developing Alzheimer's disease when in fact your confusion is caused by a medical problem such as a urinary tract infection.

End-of-Life Issues

As you age, you may find it hard to avoid thinking about death. The longer you live, the more deaths occur among your circle of family and friends. Going to funerals is something you do more often. You may spend increasing amounts of your time thinking about your life and planning for your own death.

You may have chronic illnesses that are a constant reminder of your limitations. Common long-lasting illnesses that need to be managed in older people include chronic obstructive pulmonary disease, diabetes, and hypertension. You may develop cancer and feel anxious about the side effects of treatments as well as the possibility that it will shorten your life. You may have cardiac disease and worry that your heart will develop abnormalities that could end your life or diminish the quality of your life.

As you approach the end of your life, you and your family will have important decisions to make and issues to resolve. How will you want to be treated if you become terminally ill? Would you want to be on a ventilator? Would you want to be resuscitated? Would you want to empower a family member to make decisions for you? If so, which family member? What would you like that person to do? Ideally you will discuss these topics with family members so the family knows what your wishes are.

It is highly recommended that you not only discuss plans for the end of life with family, but that you put preferences in writing. You should prepare a Living Will and Advance Directives, which tells others your preferences when you are dying (such as whether you would want to be kept alive on a ventilator). You should identify which family member you would prefer to have Durable Power of Attorney so that your business matters can be handled for you when you are no longer able to manage them yourself. You should also identify which family member you would want to have Durable Power of Healthcare Attorney, with the legal authority to make healthcare decisions for you at the end of life.

One tool that may help families focus on the issues to be discussed and decided at the end of life is a document entitled "The

Five Wishes." This document, which is available on the Internet (see resources at the end of this chapter), consists of a series of questions about how you would want to be treated at the end of your life.

Because we live in an age of advanced medical technology, it is tempting for family members to want to try everything available to prolong the life of a dying person. Letting go of a loved one is incredibly difficult. Many family issues get activated when it is time to decide how aggressively to treat a person who is terminally ill. Family members who have been less engaged may feel guilt and have difficulty accepting the upcoming loss; they may want to do anything they can to delay or avoid death of their loved one. Other family members who have watched the slow deterioration may be more able to accept when death is near. Ideally the wishes of the dying patient will be followed.

Relationships may be the most complex and difficult issues for you to address while you approach death. Did you become estranged from anyone in your family? Do you feel you have been wronged by anyone? Have you wronged another? Are you harboring anger or resentment toward any family member or friend? Can you find a way to forgive? Can you ask for forgiveness?

These issues are at the heart of the end of life. Rarely will someone who is dying wish that she had earned more money, had a more important job, or spent less time with her children. Instead, relationships determine what you will feel in your final hours. Most dying people crave contact with family and close friends and will appreciate their presence even if they are not able to fully communicate with them at the very end.

How Can the Senior Woman Tell If She Is Depressed?

Women continue to be twice as likely as men to experience depression in old age, especially "minor" depression (that is, depression not severe enough to be diagnosed as major depression). We have discussed issues that can increase a woman's risk of depression in her elder years: changes in relationships, mobility, appearance, and independence. Further, there is evidence that once a woman is postmenopausal, estrogen deficiency contributes to depressive symptoms. Women also suffer from depression longer than men, even though more women than men get treated.

Depression can be more difficult to recognize in the elderly. As a senior woman with depression, you may not even consciously realize that you are unhappy. Instead, you may feel more irritable and be annoyed easily by minor inconveniences. You may find that you no longer take pleasure in many of the activities that you previously enjoyed.

As noted earlier, appetite and sleep changes are hallmarks of depression. With age, less sleep is required—many women find that they need significantly less sleep than they did when they were younger. Sleep also becomes more fragmented with the arrival of menopause. With depression, sleep is likely to become even more disturbed. You may have difficulty falling asleep, may wake during the night repeatedly, and may wake early in the morning and not be able to get back to sleep. A minority of women with depression may sleep more than usual. Also, your appetite may either increase or decrease.

Depressed women have less energy, but decreased energy can also be the consequence of many other medical conditions and nutrition. It is important to recognize that depression may be causing the fatigue. But it is also imperative to look for other medical causes of fatigue, such as anemia and hypothyroidism.

Difficulty concentrating is a common symptom of depression, and in the elderly this symptom may be especially alarming. When you can't concentrate, you may appear to have memory deficits because you aren't able to register new information. It is easy for an older woman to fear that she is developing dementia when she starts to have problems with her memory—and if she is depressed, those memory problems may be due to depression, not to dementia.

What Can the Senior Woman Do to Improve Her Mood?

The strategies that can help senior women avoid and respond to depression are similar to strategies for people at other ages. It may feel harder at this age to take care of yourself, but this is exactly a time to increase your efforts to self-nurture. The suggestions that follow start with preventive strategies for someone who is trying to avoid depression. If these suggestions do not help, and you develop a clinical depression, treatment may be needed.

PAY ATTENTION TO YOUR DAILY SCHEDULE

- Eat and drink regularly and do not allow yourself to get too hungry.
- Make sure that you take prescription medications as directed by your doctor. You may benefit from filling up a medication box in advance, or asking someone to help you set it up. That way each day you can remember which pills to take and easily see whether you have already taken them.

GET SOCIAL INTERACTION

- Plan activities so you interact with others.
- Consider joining your local senior center, church group, book club, sewing circle, or exercise class.
- If you live around others, reach out to them and plan activities together. Seize opportunities to engage with others, such as playing cards or other games.

FIND WAYS TO EXERCISE YOUR BODY AND BRAIN

- Look for a form of exercise that you will enjoy and do consistently. Walk regularly or swim if you have access to a pool.
- Consider joining a gym, YMCA, community center, or senior center.

- Start a new hobby or return to an interest of your past. Knit, embroider, do needlework, paint, play a musical instrument, take photographs, garden, read, row a boat, make scrapbooks. Learning new things has been shown to reduce the risk of dementia.

VOLUNTEER YOUR TIME

- Donate your time by volunteering to help others. Opportunities are abundant at religious institutions, hospitals, schools, parks, and other organizations and locations.
- Think about what you enjoy and what would feel valuable to you. Helping others will give you more of a sense of meaning.

DEVELOP YOUR SPIRITUAL SIDE

- Devote time to your spirituality. This is a stage of life when worship may seem more meaningful than ever before.
- You may find companionship with others who share your faith.

SEEK PROFESSIONAL RESOURCES

- Consider therapy. Various types of individual psychotherapy can be valuable for the older woman. You may find it beneficial to review your life and relationships and construct a narrative that gives your life meaning. This is called a "life review." You may have losses that you have not fully grieved. You may have feelings of anger or resentment that you have not been able to resolve. Finding a way to forgive yourself and others for past sins can be healing.
- Think about including your family in therapy with you. Family therapy can help to identify and strengthen family

support. You may also benefit from thinking through together the various choices that will need to be made as you continue to age.

- Look into getting an evaluation to see if you could benefit from taking an antidepressant medication. If you do this, make sure that your doctor is cautious about the dosage he or she prescribes for you. It is wise to start with doses that are lower than those prescribed for younger women. Side effects may be more severe, and the benefits of treatment should be carefully weighed against that risk. Drug interactions may be more likely, since elderly women often take several medications. Ask your doctor about all the options for antidepressants. Postmenopausal women may respond better to tricyclic antidepressants than younger women (see chapter 6).
- Ask your doctor whether you might benefit from hormone replacement therapy (HRT), which is a complex topic due to its effects on multiple organ systems. Typically HRT is used only around the time of menopause, but it can also be helpful for stabilizing moods in post-menopausal women.
- Discuss with your doctor the risks and the benefits of the atypical antipsychotic group of medications, if these are recommended. These are a relatively new group of medications and include Risperdal (risperidone), Zyprexa (olanzapine), and Seroquel (quetiapine). These medications are sometimes used for their calming and sedative effects, but they have significant possible side effects, especially in the elderly. Be cautious before agreeing to take these medications.
- Investigate electroconvulsive therapy (ECT) and other alternative treatments (see chapter 6) if your depression is debilitating and does not respond to medication. ECT is sometimes recommended for elderly patients with severe depression. It may or may not be available in your community. You may be surprised at how much this treatment can

help if other treatments have been ineffective. The treatment is much more controlled today than it was in the past, but does have the side effect of causing possible memory loss for the time around the treatment itself. ECT is the single most effective treatment for depression and should be considered if other treatments do not work.

- Seek an evaluation if you are developing memory problems. Your primary care physician or a geriatric specialist can do such an evaluation for you. A variety of conditions can cause confusion and memory problems, including urinary tract infections, medication side effects, and dementia. There are multiple forms of dementia. Blood tests can identify whether you might have a reversible form of dementia. Treatments are available that may slow the progression of memory loss; medications such as Aricept (donepezil) and Namenda (memantine) may be able to slow the evolution of your dementia if it has begun. The earlier treatments begin, the more likely they are to be effective.

•

Health issues, deaths of friends and family, and loneliness can lead to low mood in the senior years. During this period of life, it is important to seek connections with others and to find coping strategies that will help you maintain your emotional balance. This can be a time of increased spirituality and an opportunity to reflect on your life. This can also be an occasion to repair relationships and to allow yourself to feel liberated from previous social constraints. There are benefits that come with aging that many people learn to appreciate, even savor.

RECOMMENDED RESOURCES

BOOKS

Joan Chittister. *The Gift of Years: Growing Older Gracefully*. New York: Blue Bridge, 2008.

Margaret Cruikshank, PhD. *Learning to Be Old: Gender, Culture, and Aging*. Lanham, MD: Rowman & Littlefield Publishers, 2013.

Ruth H. Jacobs, PhD. *Be an Outrageous Older Woman*. New York: William Morrow Paperbacks, 1997.

WEBSITE
"The Five Wishes," http://www.agingwithdignity.org/five-wishes.php

PART TWO

DISORDERS THAT CAN OCCUR
IN WOMEN OF ANY AGE

CHAPTER 6

Overcoming Depression

Amy can't seem to get herself on track. Her boyfriend recently broke up with her and she hasn't recovered. She thought he was the love of her life, and she feels lost without him. She has trouble keeping up with her college classes and has difficulty concentrating. She misses her family. She can't sleep well. She cries easily. She wonders if something is wrong with her.

Sylvia finds herself unable to recover from her sister's death a year ago. She cries almost every day and has trouble sleeping. She feels regret for lost opportunities with her sister and wishes she had spent more time with her. She's seldom hungry and has shed ten pounds in the last few months. She is lonely and wishes she had someone to talk with.

Kelly is unhappy with her job and marriage. She feels irritable at work and resentful of the assignments that are given to her. She recently left work in tears after her boss made a comment that she felt was an insult. At home she finds herself snapping at her husband, and they argue often. She doesn't understand why she feels so angry all the time, and doesn't know where to turn for help. She has started drinking every night and wonders if she is drinking too much.

Martina is the primary caregiver for her husband of 40 years who is receiving chemotherapy and radiation treatments. She has watched her husband suffer through the many side effects of his treatment. Her friends and family are supportive, but some well-meaning friends have made comments that hurt her. One friend remarked that Martina had been lucky all her life, which Martina took to mean that her friend thought it was Martina's "turn" to experience life's hardships. She feels isolated and is afraid that her husband will die. She went to see a therapist once but didn't find it helpful and can't rationalize spending more money to talk to a stranger.

•

Each of these women feels stress and some level of depression, but they feel them in different ways. Such is the case with depression—it has many faces. This chapter explores what depression is and what to look for if you think that you or a loved one might be depressed. It also describes the causes of and treatments for depression. When a person is depressed it's sometimes hard for her to believe that she will get better. With proper treatment, though, most people with depression can feel better.

What Is Depression?

The word "depression" is used by psychiatrists and other doctors when they are referring to a psychiatric illness called major depressive disorder or clinical depression. This depression is not the same as a passing mood of feeling "blue." It is safe to say that everyone at some time in his or her life feels down. In fact, feeling dejected at times is a normal and necessary part of the human experience. We need to grieve when we lose someone we love. We feel sad after the loss of a job or a relationship. Most people can tolerate such misfortunes without feeling overwhelmed, but sometimes we respond to life's stresses by developing a more serious depression. Sometimes, too, people develop clinical depression without any precipitating cause—they become depressed even though their life seems to be going along just fine.

In this chapter I use the word depression to refer to the illness that affects us in a way that creates a notably different state of mind than our usual self. It can take over the body and brain.

The cases above illustrate how depression can be felt in women of any age. Those who experience the illness of depression may lose their ability to feel pleasure. It has been described to me by one of my patients as a horror:

> Most days I wake up knowing who I am, whether I have to go to a funeral or have a fun day planned. But when I got depressed, it was as if something sucked out of me everything that *was* me, and it was replaced by something awful.

The illness of depression often goes unrecognized. It can develop slowly, without a dramatic or clearly identifiable onset. Those who experience it may not know what is happening to them. Their friends and family may notice that their behavior is different but not know why. Their doctors may not put together their symptoms and recognize that depression is what is causing their distress, especially if they focus on physical symptoms such as insomnia instead of on their mood. Some, especially adolescents and elderly people, may not even realize that they are down. Adolescents may not "act depressed"; instead, they may act and feel more irritable and may become more defiant and get in trouble more often. Some adolescents with depression become more withdrawn. Elderly people may have more physical discomforts and memory problems. Being aware of the symptoms of depression will help you recognize depression in yourself or someone you love.

Key Symptoms of Major Depression

Major depressive disorder (MDD), also called major depression, is the diagnostic term used to describe severe depression. First and foremost, someone with MDD has a profoundly different mood on a daily basis. This "black mood" is continuous, with no relief, and is distinctly different from just a "bad day." You may feel that you have no interests anymore, can no longer experience pleasure, and that nothing can cheer you. You may also become irritable and easily angered. As noted above, irritability may be the most noticeable mood change seen in adolescents with depression. Also the mood may change during the day, usually being worse in the morning. This may seem like a cruel hoax to those who think they see improvement at the end of the day, only to wake with depression back again in the morning.

People with major depression may have crying spells that are frequent and disabling. You may cry uncontrollably and find yourself bursting into tears at inappropriate times. Or you may feel a strong pressure to cry without being able to do so. Some people exert tremendous energy to put forth a superficial front of being "okay," but inside they feel great despair. They may feel hopeless as well as helpless. Tearfulness is not the key symptom for diagnosing depression, however. A more telling, and unique, symptom of major depression is having lost interest in people, things, and activities that formerly interested you or gave you pleasure.

Along with these changes in mood, a number of physical changes may occur. You may have trouble sleeping, or, less commonly, sleep more than usual. You may have trouble falling asleep and spend much time trying to make sleep come. Or, you may fall asleep only to wake up again during the night. You may also wake up early in the morning and be unable to get back to sleep. Alternatively, you may sleep more than usual and want to take multiple naps or to stay in bed most of the day.

Appetite can shift in either direction as well. For many people appetite declines. Food no longer seems appealing, and you may have to consciously remind yourself to eat. You may lose significant weight. In contrast, others find that they eat more than usual. You may turn to food for comfort or simply find that you feel hungry all the time. You may gain considerable weight. Thus it is the *change* in the former pattern of sleep and appetite that is a key symptom of depression—whether you eat more (or less) or sleep more (or less) than you did previously.

Other physical symptoms may accompany depression. Sex drive often decreases. It is common for depressed women to have no interest in sex. Usually energy decreases; you may feel tired all the time. You may also experience other bodily pains such as headaches, backaches, constipation, or stomach problems.

Depression may significantly change your activity level. It may slow you down. You may talk, speak, and move much more slowly than usual. This change can be quite noticeable to your family and friends. You may find it takes you longer than usual to complete a thought. In extreme cases, you may be so slowed that you seem almost paralyzed. Alternatively, depression may be accompanied by increased nervous energy. Some people with depression become agitated and nervous and can hardly sit still.

Your thoughts change when you become depressed. Depression may cause a big decline in self-esteem. You may feel worthless or extremely guilty for real or imagined wrongdoings. The irritability that occurs with depression can contribute to these feelings of worthlessness, especially for women whose sense of personal value depends on their caretaking roles for children or others. Negative thoughts are both a cause and an effect of depression, as will be discussed later in this chapter.

An alarming symptom you may develop is difficulty concentrating, which may cause you to feel that you are losing your mind. You may not be able to direct your attention to only one thing at a time. Instead you may go over and over your worries in your mind. You may have a hard time functioning due to your inability to focus. You may become forgetful and especially have trouble registering new information. One of the most dramatic examples of this problem with concentration that I encountered was a physician who became depressed and could not remember the security code she needed to get into her building. She was upset by her confusion and thought that she had suddenly developed dementia.

Making decisions can be hard if you are depressed. You may have trouble with even the smallest of choices, such as which batch of bananas to buy at the grocery, let alone big decisions, such as whether to get a divorce. It is usually wise, if possible, to avoid making significant life decisions while experiencing major depression. The world may look quite different once your mood improves.

The *Diagnostic and Statistical Manual of Mental Disorders*, fifth edition (*DSM-5*), the diagnostic manual for psychiatry, specifies that a person must have these conditions to be diagnosed with major depressive disorder:

(a) five or more of the symptoms listed below must be present, and

(b) they must be present for at least two weeks, and

(c) at least one of the symptoms must be depressed mood or loss of interests/pleasure.

Here is a list of the key symptoms of major depression:

- Persistent down mood lasting most of the day, nearly every day, that continues for more than a couple of weeks
- Loss of interests in usual activities or pleasure
- Sleep changes (decreased or increased)
- Appetite changes (decreased or increased) with possible weight changes
- Difficulty thinking and/or concentrating and/or indecisiveness
- Fatigue
- Overall physical and mental slowing or anxious agitation
- Feelings of worthlessness and/or excessive guilt
- Recurrent thoughts of death and possible thoughts of suicide

This last symptom, suicidal thoughts, deserves special consideration. Suicide is the most serious concern among mental health providers, and therefore mental health professionals continuously watch for suicidal thinking. If it goes unrecognized and untreated, an episode of major depression is likely to last nine months or more. It can be a frightening experience and is often accompanied by anxiety. If you have depression you may think that you will never recover. You may lose perspective. You may start to think that you do not want to live anymore and may seriously consider suicide, even if suicide was previously unthinkable.

It is a myth to think that those who speak of suicide are only issuing a "cry for help" and don't really mean it. The fact is that eight out of ten people who eventually commit suicide had let someone know about their thoughts. When a woman speaks of suicide, it is important to take her seriously. I always ask how frequently she is having such thoughts and whether she has a specific plan. If so, what is that plan? Has she begun to act on that plan? She is more at risk if she lacks a robust support system, has recent losses, and has a lethal plan. If a family member such as a sibling, parent, or grandparent has committed suicide, she is at even greater risk since there appears to be a genetic component to suicidality.

When a woman develops concrete plans for suicide, this is the time to seek help immediately. If someone is truly suicidal and on the verge of killing herself, it is considered a psychiatric emergency. Hospitalizing the suicidal person can provide safety until adequate treatment can begin.

Another myth is that asking someone about suicidal thoughts might cause damage and plant the suggestion in her mind. If you have concern about a loved one with depression, it is best to ask her directly whether she has any suicidal thoughts. If she is having such thoughts, she will likely be relieved to talk about it. And talking about it will help you to know how much in danger she might be.

A few people with severe depression develop paranoid thoughts or hallucinations. These are called *psychotic* symptoms. You could develop false beliefs, such as thinking that strangers might want to harm you. You could hear voices, see things that are not there, or smell odors that are not present. Fortunately, having these experiences does not mean that you will not get well. But it is critical that you share these symptoms with family, friends, and especially your doctor. While they can be frightening, these psychotic symptoms are likely to resolve with treatment.

Other Forms of Depression

Other forms of depressive illness can also occur, especially in women.

Atypical depression. In this variant of major depression, sleep is increased, energy is very low, and appetite is increased. Women with this type of depression may gain considerable weight. They may feel a "leaden paralysis," in which their arms or legs feel extremely heavy. They may be more sensitive to signs of rejection from others. Their mood is reactive, so that it brightens in response to actual or potentially positive events.

Persistent depressive disorder (dysthymia). This type of depression is chronic (lasts more than two years) but not as severe as major depression, and it is one and a half to three times more common in women than men. This disorder is associated with poor medical health and lower levels of social satisfaction. Poor self-esteem and feelings of hopelessness are common symptoms. Like major depression, this disorder is under-recognized and undertreated. It often occurs in conjunction with other psychiatric disorders, including major depression, anxiety disorders, and substance abuse.

Seasonal pattern of major depressive disorder, or seasonal affective disorder (SAD). SAD refers to major depression that occurs primarily during certain seasons of the year, typically in the fall and winter, with remission in spring and summer. The timing of depressive episodes is influenced by the total amount of available daylight and can be effectively treated with light therapy, using special banks of lights in specific wavelengths of light. SAD is four times more likely in women than in men. It is more common in regions that have less light, such as the Northwest and many Scandinavian countries.

Earlier in this book I discussed other variations of depression that are tied to women's reproductive systems, including the spectrum of *premenstrual mood disorders, peripartum depression* (including depression that begins during pregnancy or within four weeks after delivery), and *perimenopausal depression*. The fluctuations in hormones that occur in all women are believed to interact with other factors to make some women more vulnerable to mood problems at a variety of times in their life.

What Causes Depression?

A combination of factors can lead to depression, and anyone can become depressed, given enough stress, although some people are more vulnerable than others. Many theories exist to explain why women are more at risk for depression than men.

The categories of factors that can lead to depression are:

- Genetic
- Biological
- Psychological
- Social

GENETIC FACTORS

Our understanding of depression has changed in the last several decades. When I was in training in the 1980s, I was taught that depression was *either* "endogenous" (meaning biological and requiring medication treatment more often) *or* "reactive" (meaning related to stressors in life and not necessarily requiring medication). The implication of the old model was that endogenous depression arose from within the sufferer's physiology whereas reactive depression was presumed to be caused by something outside the sufferer. Now we have a more comprehensive combined model.

We now see major depression as an illness that can develop from a variety of causes that can occur in conjunction. Stress usually precedes depression, even in people who are genetically predisposed to it.

If depression runs in your family, you may have inherited genes that make you more susceptible to depression. You may be more at risk than others and may become depressed at a lower level of stress than others. If you have family members—grandparents, parents, aunts and uncles, siblings—who have depression or who have had depression, it's possible that you have genes making you more vulnerable to depression and it would be wise to watch for symptoms of depression in yourself.

BIOLOGICAL FACTORS

Other biological factors can cause you to become depressed. Certain medical disorders and medications are also known to increase your risk.

Depression can be *caused by another illness*, such as the following:

- Endocrine disorders: Cushing's disease, Addison's disease, diabetes mellitus, hypothyroidism, hyperthyroidism
- Collagen diseases: rheumatoid arthritis, temporal arteritis, polymyalgia rheumatica
- Chronic infections: infectious mononucleosis, hepatitis, herpes zoster, tuberculosis
- Neurological diseases: Parkinson's disease, Huntington's disease, traumatic brain injury, strokes, multiple sclerosis, Alzheimer's disease

Depression can occur *in conjunction with other illnesses*:

- Heart attack. After a heart attack, 40 to 65 percent of people develop major depression. The presence of depression increases the mortality rate from heart disease. One theory about how these illnesses interrelate is that depression may increase platelet aggregation, which is a mechanism that causes clotting to occur.
- Drug and alcohol addiction. As mentioned previously, alcohol and drug abuse often occur in conjunction with depression. Either condition can come first. Often people

with depression turn to alcohol and drugs to help themselves feel better (this is sometimes called "self-medicating"), not realizing that their depression will be worsened over the long run by alcohol and drugs. On the other hand, alcohol and drug abuse can come first and can lead to the development of depression, especially when the abuse contributes to deterioration of health, relationships, and job performance.

Depression can be *caused by treatment for another illness*:

- Steroids are notorious for their effect on mood. They can cause depression or, in some people, can create manic symptoms (discussed in chapter 9).
- Beta-blockers, medications used to treat high blood pressure, sometimes cause depression.
- Reserpine and alpha-methyldopa have been used for hypertension but both can induce depression.
- Alpha-interferon, used to treat certain cancers, multiple sclerosis, and chronic hepatitis B and C, can induce depression.

Depression in women can be caused, in part, by *hormonal changes*:

- The increased rate of depression in females starts with puberty. Hormonal cycling begins at that time, and throughout the life cycle there is evidence that times of hormonal change are associated with depression in some individuals.
- In previous chapters we discussed premenstrual, postpartum, and perimenopausal forms of depressive illness. At each of these times, women experience changing levels of female hormones that likely precipitate mood problems in those women who are vulnerable. All women experience hormonal shifts, but some women appear to be predisposed to mood problems that are triggered by the hormonal changes.

PSYCHOLOGICAL AND SOCIAL FACTORS

If there is no depression in your family, and you do not have an illness or medication that causes depression, you could still become depressed given enough stress. More women than men experience depression, and women are twice as likely to develop major depression. Many factors contribute to making women more vulnerable, including hormonal changes, our psychology, and the social roles that women play.

Psychological factors, such as negative thinking, and social factors, such as trauma or loss or relationship issues, are especially likely to lead to depression.

- Negative thinking. Depression can be *the cause* or *the result* of negative thinking. A compelling two-way interaction exists between depression and negative thinking. If depression develops due to a cause such as a medication or illness or recent loss, even if you have never been someone who has engaged in negative thinking, you are likely to begin to view the world more negatively than you did before. Conversely, if you are someone who tends to view the world more pessimistically, you are more at risk of developing depression as a result of your negative thoughts. This is an important association because it gives you a target for treatment. That is, changing your negative thoughts can help treat your depression, regardless of whether the thoughts are the cause or the result of the depression.

- Putting others first. Certain female psychological and social patterns can lead to depression. Many women put others' needs ahead of their own, to their own detriment. We take care of others. Over time we may develop resentment or feel drained and unfulfilled. We may feel too guilty to ask for time for ourselves. In an effort to be "nice," we may stifle any anger that we feel. Later that anger may leak out in the form of irritability or explosions of temper, or may be converted into depression.

- The need for connection. Connection to others is important, and women crave this bond. This concept is the basis of what has been called relational-cultural theory, developed at the Stone Center at Wellesley College. Jean Baker Miller was an early leader in identifying women's need for relationships as a strength in her 1976 book, *Toward a New Psychology of Women*, and others further developed her work. The primary tenets are that relationships with others are central to the sense of well-being in women, as important as autonomy, and that lost or threatened connections may play a role in the development of women's depression. The need for connection is normal and healthy. Absence of close bonds is a significant stressor. Losing our primary relationship, through divorce or a breakup or death of our spouse, can be especially difficult. The death of a child is one of the greatest tragedies of life and very difficult for a mother to handle, but losing children emotionally, such as when they leave home for college, is also hard. Moving to a new town is another form of loss, since it takes us away from our support system and puts us into a different environment.

A woman's friendships are central to her enjoyment of life and health and are key to her ability to be emotionally resilient when stresses do occur. A study known as the Harvard Medical School's Nurses' Health Study showed that women were less likely to have physical illness and more likely to be happy as they aged if they had more friends. This was true whether or not the women were married or had a partner.

- Stress response. Women appear to have a different response to stress than men. The "fight or flight" response describes how men typically respond to a threat: they either fight against it, or flee. For example, men may argue with their partners or their boss, or they may instead seek a new relationship or job. Women, in contrast, tend to respond to stress by following the "tend or befriend" model. Women in conflict are more inclined to gather with friends (often other women) and to tend to their children. Although these descriptions are generalizations and the difference between the genders is not absolute, these patterns of responding to stress may have a biological basis. Oxytocin is a hormone in the brain that produces relaxation and caretaking behavior. Male hormones block oxytocin release, while estrogen enhances oxytocin release. Women who are under stress and respond by talking to their friends are likely to feel calmer. When women lack connection and opportunities for friendship, they may be more vulnerable to depression.

• Trauma. Women are more likely to experience some forms of trauma, such as rape and domestic violence (although trauma certainly occurs to males as well). Depression is one of the potential consequences of these experiences. Trauma can change a woman's sense of safety in the world and in her relationships with others and can diminish her hopes for the future.

• Social expectations. Women have traditionally been expected to fulfill more subservient roles. As women in today's society achieve leadership roles, they still may find themselves marginalized or isolated in settings where male leadership predominates. At home, women adopt many homemaking roles even if they also work outside the home. In addition, in our families and our society, women are more often the primary caregivers. They find themselves caring for parents, spouses, children, and friends at times of need, and caregiving can become both physically and emotionally depleting.

What Can You Do If You Think You May Be Depressed?

If you suspect that you or your friend or family member might be depressed there are a number of strategies that I would recommend.

GET A PHYSICAL EXAMINATION

If you think you might be depressed, this would be a good time to have an overall physical examination and lab tests. If you do not have a primary care physician, ask your friends to recommend someone, or check with your insurance company to learn which doctors are in your network. Tell your doctor that you have been feeling down and describe in detail what you are experiencing.

The symptoms of thyroid disease mimic the symptoms of depression and can be easily mistaken for depression. Ask your doctor to check your thyroid hormone levels, since the thyroid is the most common medical cause of depression and any imbalance can be corrected if the thyroid is found to be either overactive or underactive. Thyroid function tests are not routinely ordered by most primary care physicians, so make sure this test is included in your lab work. If thyroid disease is present but is not discovered, other treatments for depression are unlikely to work. Other diseases such as anemia can mimic depression as well and may need to be treated directly.

EXERCISE

Exercise has been demonstrated to be an effective treatment for mild to moderate levels of depression. It really works, is free, and is available to everyone!

- Take a walk around your neighborhood, choose the stairs rather than the elevator, or engage in another form of sport.
- Buy a bicycle and ride around your neighborhood.
- Join a health club, which has the additional benefit of being surrounded by others who are also seeking to be healthy.

For those who have never been athletic or haven't developed the exercise habit, the thought of starting to exercise may not sound appealing. It is hard to change your behavior. Exercise for the sake of exercise can be hard to force yourself to do. But consider this: exercise can really make you feel better emotionally. Any day that you are feeling down or anxious, just taking a walk or exercising at the gym can boost your mood. Try it and pay attention to how you feel. Give yourself a pat on the back for making an effort, and give yourself time to start feeling better. Start planning your days around time to exercise. You will see the benefits.

PRACTICE GOOD SLEEP HYGIENE

Restful sleep is important for your overall emotional well-being, and poor sleep may contribute to depression. Many people with depression suffer with insomnia. They have a hard time falling asleep or they wake up during the night and struggle to get back to sleep. Early-morning awakening is a common symptom of depression. If you are having sleep problems, there are a number of things you can do to improve your sleep.

- Avoid drinking alcoholic beverages near bedtime.
- Avoid excessive caffeine intake from coffee, tea, chocolate, and other caffeine-heavy foods, or cut caffeine from your diet entirely. Caffeine is an obvious stimulant, but there are other stimulants that interfere with sleep, such as exercise.
- Exercise early in the day, not close to bedtime.
- Develop a sleep routine, which most people find helpful. You can create a routine at bedtime that avoids stimulation: for example, take a warm bath or read a book that you know will not affect you emotionally or otherwise keep you awake. Consume foods high in the amino acid tryptophan as a bedtime snack, such as warm milk and bananas. Allow yourself enough time to sleep: put yourself to bed early enough so that you have time to get the sleep you need. Get up at the same time every morning.

- Sleep in a cool, dark, quiet room without a visible clock, in a comfortable bed. If you wake up at night and cannot get back to sleep, get up and leave the bedroom, read or do some quiet activity until you are sleepy again. Do not lie in bed and try to force yourself to sleep.
- Beware of watching television or working on a computer or any kind of tablet or smartphone in the bedroom, since the light from the screen has been shown to be stimulating.
- Avoid daytime napping, which may interfere with your body's need for sleep at night.
- Consider sleep medication, but only after trying other remedies. There are medications to induce and maintain sleep, but before you use a medication try avoiding stimulants and developing a sleep routine, as suggested above. It is far better to train your body to respond to a routine, and to avoid the possibility of becoming physically or psychologically dependent on any drug to help you sleep. If you are exhausted from lack of sleep, however, see your doctor and consider using a sleep medication for a short time. Sleep medications include over-the-counter options such as the hormone melatonin and the antihistamine benadryl, and prescription medications that your doctor may recommend to you for sleep. See table 1 for a summary of sleep agents. Most of the medications in this table are meant for short-term use only. Three of them (Desyrel, Remeron, and Silenor) are sedating antidepressants that are sometimes given at low doses to aid with sleep.
- Obtain a sleep study. Talk to your doctor if you have persistent sleep problems. You may benefit from a sleep study to find out whether you have a sleep disorder. Disorders such as sleep apnea and restless legs syndrome can be diagnosed with a sleep study, and your sleep may become much more restful if these disorders are treated.

TABLE 1   *Commonly Used Prescription Sleep Medications*

Brand name	Generic name	Recommended dose range*
Ambien	zolpidem	5–10 mg (5 mg for women)
Lunesta	eszopiclone	2–3 mg
Sonata	zaleplon	5–20 mg
Rozerem	ramelteon	8 mg
Desyrel	trazodone	25–100 mg
Remeron	mirtazapine	7.5 mg
Silenor	doxepin	3–6 mg

*As of 2015.

EAT NUTRITIOUS FOOD

You will feel better emotionally if you eat a healthy diet. Many people who are feeling depressed neglect their own needs, including the need to eat well. You may have difficulty finding the motivation to take good care of yourself, but try to focus on eating well, it is such an important ingredient for mental health.

- Portion size matters. Eating well includes eating appropriate portions of food—enough to satisfy your hunger but not leave you feeling stuffed. Eat several small meals a day.
- Take time to savor your meals by eating slowly, preferably with others.
- Strive for balance. Make up your mind that you are going to eat a balanced diet, with protein, fat, carbohydrates, fiber, vitamins, and minerals. Choose whole grains instead of white flour, white rice, and refined sugar. Limit saturated fats, found in red meat and whole milk, and curb trans fats, found in fried foods and processed foods. Eat lots of fresh fruits and vegetables. The website www.choosemyplate.gov is a gold mine of helpful advice about how to eat a satisfying and healthy diet and provides charts of recommended quantities.
- Pay attention to your intake of calcium. It is recommended that you consume 1000 mg per day of calcium, or

1200 mg if you are over age 50. It is best to obtain your calcium from natural sources, such as dairy products, leafy green vegetables, and beans, rather than from supplements (calcium pills or chews). Greek yogurt is an excellent source of calcium, with 450 mg per serving. Do not eat more than 2000 mg per day, since too much calcium may lead to kidney stones and other problems. Ask your doctor about your specific calcium needs.

- Watch your Vitamin D levels. Vitamin D is another important dietary component. Your doctor may measure your vitamin D level to see if it is adequate. Research shows that vitamin D can benefit your mood. As with calcium, too much vitamin D can be harmful. Seek guidance from your doctor about whether you might need a vitamin D supplement in your diet.

FIND CONFIDING RELATIONSHIPS

Finding someone to talk to about your problems has been shown to be protective against depression and can be healing. It fits with the relational theory that we discussed in the previous section. Women especially need to talk to an understanding listener. We need connection.

- Avoid isolation. Many women with depression isolate themselves. Over time a married woman may pull away from other friends and spend most of her time with her husband. If she develops conflict with her husband, she has nowhere to turn for support. Many women serve in a caregiver role for others, leaving less time for confiding relationships. Depression itself may cause her to want to withdraw from others.
- Find supportive companions. Think of family and friends who could be supportive. Look for empathic listeners as well as for people whose company you enjoy. Put a priority on making time for being with your confidante. Plan some walks or lunches or dinners where you can have leisurely,

private conversations. Don't wait for others to initiate the activities—issue the invitation yourself.

- Be an empathic listener. How can you be supportive to someone else with depression? The key is to focus on empathic listening, not on coming up with solutions for your friend or family member. Give her time to talk and reflect. Suggest activities that you can do together (such as taking a walk or having a meal), and express sincere interest in how she is doing. Ask her open-ended questions that cannot be answered with a simple yes or no, and let her tell you what she is thinking and feeling. The simple act of listening is a special gift to someone with depression.

RESTRUCTURE YOUR TIME

Managing the time in our day is a challenge for all of us. When we are depressed, this can seem much more difficult. At one extreme are women who overschedule their time, who run from one activity to another with no time for themselves. Mothers of young children and working mothers, for example, may find it difficult to find even a few minutes to themselves. At the other extreme are women who are so depressed that they can barely get out of bed, they isolate themselves from others, and they are unable to effectively plan and use their time.

Women at both ends of this spectrum can benefit from giving thought to how they structure their time each day. For the overscheduled woman, this may mean finding something to say "no" to.

- Can you afford to drop off a committee?
- Can you ask another mother or your partner to share some tasks with you?
- Can you find a way to modify your work schedule so that your days are not so busy?
- Can you plan to take a break during your week to have lunch with a friend or have time for yourself?

The woman at the other end of the spectrum may benefit from pushing herself to create a plan for each day. Everyone needs a reason to get out of bed in the morning.

- Create small goals for each day and write them down (as in a monthly calendar). This can be motivating and can help you to "get out of your own head."
- Plan to meet a friend for coffee, lunch, dinner, or a walk; it will improve your connections as well as give structure to your day.
- Make a commitment to volunteer regularly, this will provide you with social connections as well as a sense of making a meaningful contribution to others.

REDUCE OR STOP USING ALCOHOL

Many depressed women turn to alcohol for some relief. They may experience temporary improvement in their mood but not realize that alcohol is making their depression worse. You don't have to be an "alcoholic" for alcohol to make you more depressed. Stopping your alcohol use can be an important step toward improving your mood. Whether alcohol use comes before or after depression, your mood is likely to improve if you stop drinking. I have been impressed over the years with how many of my patients with depression improve after they stop drinking. Conversely, those who continue to drink are unlikely to respond to other treatments.

KEEP A JOURNAL

Writing in a journal can help improve your mood. It gives you a safe way to get your thoughts and feelings out and channels them in a more positive direction. Anyone can keep a journal— you don't need to be a great writer for journaling to be effective. You can write as little or as much as you want.

You can use your journal to improve your mood by simply writing down each day several things for which you are grateful. Writing down what you pray for or wish for may be helpful, too.

Journaling is much more likely to be useful to you if you include positive redirection. The psychologist Martin Seligman (see the resources at the end of this chapter) and others have studied and written about journaling as part of what they call the positive psychology method. Keeping a journal can also help you to gain perspective on your emotional journey. Over time you will find patterns in your moods and life.

There is no single or correct way to write in a journal. You can choose to journal daily or even more frequently, or you may journal only when you feel the urge. Some people use their journals for creative writing, such as poetry. Save your journals. You may be surprised when you look back at the concerns you had in past times, and you may learn about yourself and your thought processes.

MAKE TIME FOR SPIRITUAL PRACTICES

Spiritual practices are central in the lives of many people. I regularly ask women with depression about their spirituality and its role in their lives. Many say that they found meaning in church activities or other worship, but that they quit going or no longer enjoy it. It is common for people with depression to detach from religious activities as part of the overall withdrawal from others. If this is true for you, think through whether you want to re-engage with your spiritual community. You may not follow a formal spiritual practice but may be searching for more meaning in your life. You may also benefit from exploring alternative spiritual practices such as yoga and meditation. You may find that your life feels more complete if you can devote time to your spirituality.

SEEK MEANING IN YOUR ACTIVITIES

Meaningful work can be protective against depression. We have a basic need to feel that our lives have a purpose. It is a good idea to occasionally review your choices and consider other ways to increase your sense of meaning. There are many ways to accomplish this.

- Do volunteer work.
- Give support to friends and family.
- Participate in charitable activities.
- Work in a fulfilling job.

CONSIDER TALK THERAPY

Talk therapy (psychotherapy) is an effective treatment for depression. For mild to moderate depression, it can be as effective as medication. For many people who suffer from major depression, the ideal treatment is to combine therapy and medication.

There are several forms of therapy and a variety of professionals who can provide therapy to you. You could see a psychiatrist, psychologist, social worker, or a therapist with other expertise such as a marriage and family counselor. The key ingredient that leads to successful treatment is a good relationship with your therapist, not what type of therapy. If you do not find that therapy is helping, do not give up. You may find better rapport with someone else, or another therapist's approach might be a better fit for your needs.

Most therapists use a blend of therapeutic approaches. Few therapists practice only one approach, except perhaps in academic centers that are teaching new therapists. Most therapists utilize skills from various schools of therapy as they seem useful.

- *Cognitive behavioral therapy* (CBT) is one of the best-studied forms of therapy and has been demonstrated repeatedly to be an effective treatment for depression. Aaron Beck developed this approach in the 1960s, based on the observation that many people with depression have errors in their thinking and beliefs that lead them to feel depressed. They may make false assumptions or over-generalize. They may have "automatic thoughts" that are negative and discouraging, without even realizing that they are having them. For example, they may think "I always lose" or "I am useless" or "no one wants to talk to me." Such thoughts tend to worsen the mood and may lead to behaviors such as withdrawal and isolation that can lead to more depression. CBT relies on helping the patient develop thoughts that are more adaptive. It helps identify specific errors in thinking and teaches more flexible ways of thinking.

- *Dialectical behavior therapy (DBT)* is a cognitively based group therapy approach that focuses on coping skills.
- *Mindfulness-based cognitive therapy (MBCT)* is a newer version of cognitive therapy that also includes an ancient form of meditation called being "mindful." MBCT aims to interrupt automatic thought processes and allow more reflective responses. When you practice mindfulness, you become aware of your incoming thoughts and feelings but learn not to attach or react to them. Meditation helps to develop mindfulness. MBCT is based on the mindfulness-based stress reduction program of Jon Kabat-Zinn, which has been extensively studied and found to be effective for depression, pain control, and other problems.
- *Positive psychology* was developed in recent years and championed by Martin Seligman and others. This approach focuses on nurturing strengths and fostering resilience rather than concentrating only on emotional problems. It includes a number of interventions that aim to increase positive emotions and make life more fulfilling.
- *Psychodynamic therapy*, also known as *insight-oriented psychotherapy*, is another major approach that is based on the work of Sigmund Freud, Carl Jung, and others. The basis for this approach is the theory that relationships from the past influence present behavior. Unconscious conflicts develop early in life and drive behaviors. Patterns are established in earlier periods of life that may repeat and influence the present. The therapist helps the patient to gain insight into these conflicts and patterns so she can make healthier choices.
- *Psychoanalysis* refers to the original method of psycho-dynamic psychotherapy developed by Sigmund Freud, a lengthy process in which the therapist looks for unconscious

patterns developed since childhood. This approach requires that the patient lie on a couch several times per week and talk about what is on her mind. This approach may allow patients to develop insight and change patterns of behavior.

- *Interpersonal therapy* is a well-studied form of therapy found to be effective for depression. Gerald Klerman and Myrna Weissman developed it. It emphasizes social relationships in the present rather than the impact of the past. Unresolved grief, role disputes, role transitions, and interpersonal deficits are specific areas of focus.
- *Couples therapy* is sometimes helpful for women with depression, since relationship issues may be intertwined with depression. Couples often have more conflict when one or both partners are depressed, and it can be hard to know whether the depression or relationship problems came first. Depression causes irritability and loss of enthusiasm that can result in relationship conflict, and conflict is unsettling and can cause depression. Usually it is best to wait until one or both partners' depression has improved before starting couples therapy, since this form of treatment can become more challenging as issues get confronted.
- *Family therapy* can help, especially if there are family members who may be key to the recovery process. If you have conflicts with specific family members, it may be useful to include them in treatment and address issues directly. Involving family members also can expand understanding and strengthen support.
- *Group therapy* may reduce the isolation seen with depression. You can learn from others who have experienced similar struggles, as well as learning from the therapist.

GET AN EVALUATION FOR ANTIDEPRESSANT MEDICATION

Antidepressant medication can be very effective for relieving the symptoms of major depression or persistent depressive disorder. Your doctor may recommend that you begin an antidepressant, often in combination with psychotherapy. A number of medications can be prescribed by a psychiatrist or your primary care physician.

Some people fear taking antidepressants because of the false belief that they may become addicted. Antidepressants are not addicting, but they should not be stopped abruptly. Instead, when you are ready to stop the antidepressant, you should taper it slowly, in consultation with the prescriber. Usually if an antidepressant is prescribed for a single episode of major depression, the recommendation is that the medication be continued for at least a year after it begins to work and then be discontinued slowly, and ideally at a time when stressors are reduced. If you have experienced more than two episodes of major depression, then the typical recommendation is to consider staying on the antidepressant as a preventative measure. Follow-up studies have shown that, if the medication is stopped, a recurrence of depression is likely in a person who has had more than two episodes of depression.

A variety of antidepressants are available. They differ in terms of their mechanism and side effects. Table 2 summarizes the drug class, brand names, and recommended dose ranges of the most commonly used antidepressants. Table 3 summarizes the same information for older antidepressants that are still in use. In both tables I have listed both the commonly known brand name for each drug and the equivalent generic name. Your doctor, pharmacy, or insurance company may substitute the generic for the brand name drug; generics and brand name drugs usually have about the same effectiveness.

In general, the best predictor for which antidepressant will be effective for you is whether the same antidepressant worked for you before. If a family member has responded well to a particular antidepressant, it will likely be effective for you (just as the vulnerability to depression runs in families, so does the response to specific drugs). Since there is no evidence that any one medication is superior to the others, I do not prefer a specific antidepressant. My goal is to find the right "match" for each individual, and to give the medication enough time to work. You may feel some benefit within the first week or so, but you should wait four to six weeks for an adequate trial of the medication at a given dose.

- SSRIs. The selective serotonin reuptake inhibitors (SSRIs) are the most commonly used antidepressants. These medications act on the serotonin system of neurotransmitters (chemicals) in the brain by blocking reuptake (absorption) of serotonin back into the presynaptic nerve cell.
- SNRIs. Another group of medications, known as the serotonin norepinephrine reuptake inhibitors (SNRIs), block the reabsorption of both serotonin and norepinephrine in the brain.
  - Blocking reabsorption results in increased levels of neurotransmitters in the synapse (gap between nerve cells).
  - Another mechanism for both SSRIs and SNRIs is that the postsynaptic receptors for these chemicals are "down-regulated" by antidepressants, meaning that the number and sensitivity of receptors that had become "up-regulated" due to the deficiency of neurotransmitter are reduced back to more normal levels.
  - An additional current theory is that neurons (cells) in the depressed brain benefit from the release of "neurotrophic" (growth) factors induced by antidepressant drugs.
- Older medications. Antidepressants developed before the SSRIs were created are not used frequently today, due primarily to safety and side effect concerns. An overdose of tricyclic antidepressants can be lethal. They also slow your cardiac conduction so the electrocardiogram (EKG) must be monitored before and after treatment. The monoamine oxidase inhibitors (MAOIs) potentially have lethal interactions with other drugs and certain foods. These medications can still be of benefit for some individuals but should be used with caution.

Unfortunately, no antidepressant medication works immediately. Typically it takes up to four to six weeks at the therapeutic

TABLE 2   *Commonly Used Antidepressant Medications*

Brand name	Generic name	Recommended dose range*
SELECTIVE SEROTONIN REUPTAKE INHIBITORS (SSRIs)		
Celexa	citalopram	20–40 mg/day
Lexapro	escitalopram	10–20 mg/day
Luvox, Luvox CR	fluvoxamine	50–300 mg/day (100–300 mg/day CR)
Paxil, Paxil CR	paroxetine	20–60 mg/day (25–75 mg/day CR)
Prozac, Sarafem, Prozac Weekly	fluoxetine	20–80 mg/day (90 mg/week Prozac weekly)
Zoloft	sertraline	50–200 mg/day
SEROTONIN NOREPINEPHRINE REUPTAKE INHIBITORS (SNRIs)		
Cymbalta	duloxetine	40–60 mg/day
Effexor	venlafaxine	75–225 mg/day
Pristiq	desvenlafaxine	50–100 mg/day
Fetzima	levomilnacipran	40–120 mg/day
OTHER ANTIDEPRESSANTS		
Desyrel	trazodone	150–600 mg/day
Remeron	mirtazapine	15–45 mg/day at night
Viibryd	vilazodone	40 mg/day
Wellbutrin, Budeprion, Wellbutrin & Budeprion SR, Wellbutrin & Budeprion XL	bupropion	225–450 mg/day (200–450 mg/day for Wellbutrin & Budeprion SR; 150–450 mg/day for Wellbutrin & Budeprion XL)
Brintellix	vortioxetine	10–20 mg/day

*As of 2015.

dose (the dose that "works") for the medication to help you. If you are not feeling better by then, your doctor may increase your dose. If side effects occur, they most likely appear at the beginning of treatment and may decrease within a week or two. It is important to keep taking an antidepressant long enough for it to work. The most common reasons for antidepressants to be ineffective are that they were either not given long enough or not given at a suf-

TABLE 3   *Older Antidepressants*

Brand name	Generic name	Recommended dose range*
TRICYCLIC ANTIDEPRESSANTS		
Anafranil	clomipramine	100–250 mg/day
Asendin	amoxapine	200–300 mg/day
Elavil	amitriptyline	25–150 mg/day
Ludiomil	maprotiline	75–150 mg/day
Norpramin	desipramine	100–200 mg/day
Pamelor, Aventyl	nortriptyline	75–150 mg/day
Sinequan	doxepin	75–150 mg/day
Tofranil	imipramine	50–150 mg/day
Vivactil	protriptyline	15–40 mg/day
MONOAMINE OXIDASE INHIBITORS (MAOIs)		
Marplan	isocarboxazid	40–60 mg/day
Nardil	phenelzine	45–75 mg/day
Parnate	tranylcypromine	30–60 mg/day

*As of 2015.

ficient dose. You need adequate time on the antidepressant at a therapeutic dose to be able to judge whether a specific antidepressant works for you or not. Don't stop your medication once you start it without discussing side effects and mood changes with your doctor. If changes are needed, your doctor will slowly taper your medication.

I start women with a lower dose of an antidepressant than I prescribe for a man. Many women are sensitive to side effects (such as nausea and diarrhea), especially if they also experience anxiety with their depression. I have seen many women stop a medication after only one dose because they were concerned about the side effects. If you stop too soon, the medication is not given a chance to work. By gradually increasing the dose, these women have the opportunity to adapt to the medication. Side effects usually diminish over time, so this "start low, go slow" strategy helps many women to gently adapt to a medication.

The side effects of each antidepressant vary with the individual. It is fascinating to me to see how one woman may find a medication like Paxil to be sedating while another finds the same medication to be energizing. I often tell my patients to take these medications at bedtime if they are sedating, or in the morning if they are stimulating. For the majority of people, the side effects of the antidepressants, if any, occur at the beginning of treatment (and are less likely if the dose is started low and increased slowly as just described). The most common side effects of SSRIs are nausea and diarrhea. Sexual dysfunction can occur, including decreased sexual interest and/or inability to achieve an orgasm. Wellbutrin (bupropion) is less likely to cause sexual dysfunction and is sometimes prescribed together with an SSRI to treat the sexual side effect. Viibryd (vilazodone) and Brintellix (vortioxetine) also may have fewer sexual side effects.

Side effects of SNRIs include nausea, dry mouth, dizziness, sedation, insomnia, constipation, excessive sweating, agitation, or anxiety. Longer-acting forms of SNRIs reduce these side effects. The SNRI Effexor (venlafaxine) may increase blood pressure (especially in higher doses, above 150 mg per day), so blood pressure should be checked periodically.

Some antidepressants can cause you to gain weight, which varies depending on the person and medication. An increase in appetite can indicate improvement in mood for women who had lost weight due to depression. Other women may eat more as a symptom of their depression. If weight gain becomes an issue, this is something that should be discussed with your doctor.

Another potential consequence of treatment with antidepressants is that suicidal thinking may worsen. There is controversy about how much this is a side effect of treatment, since suicidal thinking is also a core symptom of depression. The FDA now requires a "black box" warning on antidepressants to give caution about this possibility, especially when antidepressants are given to children, adolescents, or young adults. It is important to keep a watch out for suicidal thinking in anyone with depression, whether or not she is taking an antidepressant, and to regularly ask whether such thoughts are occurring.

The symptoms of depression that are described earlier in this chapter are all likely to improve over time after treatment with the right antidepressant and dosage. Your sleep and appetite are likely to return to normal. Your energy, concentration, and interest in activities should get better. Dose and combinations of medications may need to be adjusted in order to attain full recovery.

After starting antidepressant treatment, individuals who have bipolar disorder may develop symptoms of mania (see chapter 9). Symptoms include increased energy, decreased need for sleep, talking much faster than usual, and reckless behavior. This is a well-known risk but is often a surprise, since bipolar disorder may only be discovered after treatment for an initial depressive episode. If it is already known that you have bipolar disorder, you need to be treated with a mood stabilizing medication *before* an antidepressant is prescribed, to protect you from developing mania. If you do develop manic symptoms, your doctor is likely to ask you to stop the antidepressant and to start a mood stabilizer medication.

WEIGH THE BENEFIT OF ADDING OTHER MEDICATIONS

Adding another type of medication may increase the effectiveness of antidepressants. One strategy combines an antidepressant with an atypical antipsychotic such as Abilify (aripiprazole), Zyprexa (olanzapine), Risperdal (risperidone), or Seroquel (quetiapine) (see table 8 in chapter 9). While these medications may be helpful, they also come with their own set of side effects including weight gain, sedation, lipid elevation, and increase in prolactin release. Other medications that are sometimes used with antidepressants include thyroid hormone or lithium. Thyroid hormone may be helpful even for women who do not have hypothyroidism. Your blood levels of lithium should be monitored if you are taking lithium (see chapter 9 on bipolar disorder).

For women who are approaching menopause (that is, women who are perimenopausal), estrogen may improve mood when given alone or in conjunction with antidepressants. Estrogen should be combined with progesterone for women who still have their uterus, due to the risk of "unopposed" estrogen causing cancer of the uterus. Estrogen can be given without progesterone for women who have had a hysterectomy, and this may be beneficial since progesterone can diminish the mood benefit from estrogen. Estrogen has some benefit by itself for treating depression in perimenopausal women, and estrogen may also improve the effectiveness of antidepressants in perimenopausal depression.

After menopause, the benefit of estrogen for the mood is less clear. When given alone at this stage, estrogen has not been shown to be beneficial for depression. When given in conjunction with antidepressants, estrogen may augment their effect, but research on this question has been inconsistent. As previously mentioned, addition of progesterone to hormone replacement therapy reduces the benefit from estrogen. Antidepressants have been shown to be helpful for women with depression who have not responded to hormone replacement therapy. Antidepressants may also effectively treat hot flashes and other symptoms of menopause, so they may be an alternative to hormone replacement therapy for some women. Women who are treated with estrogen-blocking medications (such as those used for breast cancer chemotherapy) sometimes find that their mood worsens due to this estrogen blockade.

Occasionally an antidepressant becomes less effective over time, but why this happens is not fully understood. If this occurs, your doctor is likely to increase the dose. If you continue to have a poor response, it is often best to switch to a different antidepressant altogether. Later you may benefit from starting the original medication again. The circumstances of your life may also contribute to a return of depressive symptoms, and these should be considered as well when a medication appears to stop working.

St. John's wort (Hypericum perforatum) is a dietary supplement available without a prescription that has been touted as a treatment for mild depression, but this herb is not FDA-approved and does not have clear evidence of benefit. Since it is not regulated by the FDA, there is no guarantee about the amount of active ingredient or the safety of its production. In addition, it can interact with other medications. Be sure to discuss with your doctor if you do choose to take this or any other herbal remedy.

There is some suggestion that omega-3 fatty acids (found in fish oil) may help depression, but evidence has been mixed. In addition, s-adenosylmethionine (SAMe) is another naturally occurring compound that has been studied for possible use for depression, but there is no evidence for clear benefit. The FDA approves neither of these alternative treatments.

In general, I urge caution before using complementary and alternative medications for two reasons: the absence of clear evidence for their benefit and the lack of rigorous oversight for their production.

LOOK INTO OTHER BIOLOGICAL TREATMENTS

* *Phototherapy.* Seasonal affective disorder (SAD) was mentioned earlier as a mood disorder that is more common at certain seasons of the year, especially winter, when there is less light. Those who live in regions of the world with less daylight, like the Pacific Northwest with its rain and cloud cover and Scandinavian countries with their long nights, are more likely to develop SAD than people in areas with more sunlight such as Florida. Phototherapy is a treatment approach that has been found to be helpful for prevention and treatment of SAD. Phototherapy treatment simply requires you to sit in front of a bright light box each day. In clinical trials the duration of exposure needed has been found to vary between 15 minutes and an hour, and also depends on the brightness of the equipment that is used. Light boxes are comparatively cheap, and your insurance may cover the cost of buying one. This approach can be used instead of or in addition to other treatments. Phototherapy is not used by itself as a treatment for major depression, but it can help the moodiness that comes to

some when the days start to shorten. Its side effects are infrequent, consisting of possible eyestrain, headaches, and sleep disturbance. Some people find it helps in just a week.

- *Transcranial Magnetic Stimulation (TMS)* is a relatively new treatment approach that has received considerable attention in recent years. It can enhance the effectiveness of antidepressants. It can be done in a doctor's office and does not require sedation or anesthesia. The patient remains conscious during the treatment.

TMS treatment involves holding a magnetic coil at a specific location next to your head. This coil stimulates nerve cells in a portion of your brain that is thought to play a role in mood regulation. The coil releases brief magnetic pulses into the brain. When the pulses are given in rapid succession, the technique is called repetitive TMS or rTMS. You receive this treatment every day for several weeks. Risks of rTMS include rare seizures and fainting, but overall this treatment has few side effects and is well tolerated. The FDA approved TMS in 2008 for the treatment of depression in adults when at least one antidepressant has not worked. It is generally considered to be less effective, but safer, than ECT (discussed below). Medicare approved TMS in 2012, and other insurance carriers may approve coverage on a case-by-case basis.

- *Vagal nerve stimulation (VNS)* is another recently developed treatment for depression that may be tried if other approaches have not worked. A "stimulator" is surgically implanted in the upper left chest under the collarbone, similar to placing a very small pacemaker there. Then another device which stimulates the vagal nerve is placed in the neck. Once the surgical implant has been done, a psychiatrist can monitor and adjust the VNS device. The side effects include cough and hoarseness, usually only during the 30 seconds that the stimulator is on. In 2005 the FDA approved the use of VNS for treatment-resistant depression.

- *Electroconvulsive treatment (ECT)* is the most effective treatment for severe depression. Although it is approximately 90 percent effective, it is usually reserved for patients who have not improved by taking antidepressants. ECT requires anesthesia, and a specialist must administer the treatment. There is risk of memory impairment as a side effect. If memory is lost, it is usually only the memory of the events immediately before and after the ECT treatment.

    ECT treatment has been controversial over the years. The way media (such as books and movies) portrayed ECT led to much fear of this treatment. Over the years, however, treatment guidelines were developed, and the current application of this treatment is much safer and less traumatic than in the past.

- *Deep brain stimulation (DBS)* is the newest treatment for severe major depression. Helen Mayberg pioneered DBS to treat depression that has not responded to other approaches. Although DBS is still in the experimental phase (it has not yet been approved by the FDA), it holds great promise. After an electrode is implanted into a specific area of the brain, a device can then send electrical pulses to this area. DBS has also been used successfully for some time for other disorders such as Parkinson's disease. It is a more invasive approach, because it requires a surgical intervention into the brain itself, but its use for treatment-resistant depression can cause impressive mood improvement for individuals who are severely depressed and not helped by multiple other treatment efforts.

•

Depression can be frightening and can rob life of its pleasures. For the majority of people who become depressed, a combination of factors led to the development of the depression and a combination of approaches will most likely bring relief. Everything from medications and counseling to spirituality and social changes can help. There is much evidence that depression is under-recognized and undertreated. Although our treatments are imperfect and not everyone may benefit from them, the field of psychiatry has come a long way and there are many reasons to be optimistic. We can hope that the explosion in knowledge in recent years about the functioning of the brain will translate into more effective treatments.

RECOMMENDED RESOURCES

BOOKS

Judith S. Beck, PhD. *Cognitive Behavior Therapy: Basics and Beyond*, 2d ed. New York: Guilford Press, 2011.

David Burns, MD. *Feeling Good: The New Mood Therapy*. New York: Harper Collins Publishers, 2008.

William J. Knaus, EdD. *The Cognitive Behavioral Workbook for Depression*. Oakland, CA: New Harbinger Publications, 2012.

Francis Mark Mondimore, MD. *Depression: The Mood Disease*, 3rd edition. Baltimore: Johns Hopkins University Press, 2006.

Mark Williams, PhD, John Teasdale, PhD, Zindel Segal, PhD, and Jon Kabat-Zinn, PhD. *The Mindful Way through Depression: Freeing Yourself from Chronic Unhappiness*. New York: Guilford Press, 2007.

WEBSITES

For Depression and Bipolar Support Alliance: www.dbsalliance.org/
For National Alliance on Mental Illness: www.nami.org/

CHAPTER 7

Calming Your Nerves When You Are Anxious

Jasmine is feeling very uneasy. She has just walked into a situation that scares her and is so nervous that she feels like jumping out of her skin. Her hands tremble and her heart races. Waves of fear flood her senses, creating feelings that are hard to endure. She cannot find a way to feel calm. She wonders if other people can tell how anxious she is feeling.

What Is Anxiety?

The good news about anxiety is that it serves a purpose in our lives if we can harness and control it. Henry Ward Beecher called it "the soul's signal for rallying." Without it, we might never be motivated for any productive activity. The challenge is to find a way to have enough but not too much anxiety so that it can fuel us without overwhelming us.

Jasmine's experience illustrates one of several ways we can experience anxiety. Everyone feels some degree of fear and anxiety at times, and it can range from mild to severe. Mild anxiety can be helpful. In school, it can motivate you to study. Anxiety about getting fired can motivate you to show up for work on time and do your job well. Anxiety about a performance as a musician or actor can inspire you to rehearse more intensively. Anxiety can be a good thing when it is not excessive and can provide a driving force for a more fulfilling life.

In contrast, severe anxiety—what Jasmine feels—is disabling. As with depression, women are twice as likely as men to experience anxiety disorders, and rates of women who have severe anxiety appear to be increasing. There are several types of anxiety: panic attacks, obsessive-compulsive disorder, phobias, and others. Anxiety disorders may also coexist with depression. In this chapter you will hear the stories of several women and learn to recognize the various anxiety disorders. Most importantly you will learn what you can do if you struggle with anxiety.

GENERALIZED ANXIETY DISORDER (GAD)

Alice is a worrier. All her life she has been high-strung and it is hard for her to stay calm in the face of stress. Sometimes she gets headaches, and when things get more intense she may get a stomachache. She has trouble relaxing and enjoying herself. She has trouble sleeping. Her friends call her a "worry wart." She realizes that she worries excessively, but she cannot stop herself.

Alice suffers from a pervasive form of anxiety that has affected her all her life. She was likely born with an anxious temperament. We now know that some babies display higher levels of irritability and are harder to soothe. This inborn temperament often persists through life.

Those who suffer from anxiety may not be able to soothe themselves when they encounter the stresses that are inevitable in all our lives. They react. They may get flooded with a very unpleasant feeling and think that they cannot stand to go on like that. The ability to regulate emotions is a skill: some women naturally are extremely good at this and can nurture others easily. In contrast, other women find stressors that might seem minor to some to be overwhelming. This condition is called generalized anxiety disorder (GAD).

Those who suffer from GAD feel anxious and worried almost all the time. Their concerns shift as various stressors occur, but they are rarely able to feel at peace. They may have a variety of physical symptoms such as:

- Restlessness or tension
- Difficulty concentrating
- Fatigue
- Irritability
- Muscle tension
- Difficulty sleeping

Treatments for anxiety will be addressed later in this chapter. It's worth saying now, though, that people who have GAD should be careful about beginning a regimen of medications that are known to be addicting, due to the long-term nature of GAD.

PANIC DISORDER WITH AGORAPHOBIA

Cathy is the manager for a small business. One day last month while at work she suddenly felt flooded with fear. She couldn't identify what brought this feeling on. She became panicked, and for about ten minutes she thought she was about to die. She wanted to escape. Her heart raced and she felt it pounding in her chest. She felt dizzy and lightheaded. Afterwards she felt shaken and was left with great fear that this could happen again. Since then, she has had several more such attacks. Now she is preoccupied with fear that this horrible feeling will come back. She is starting to avoid social activities out of fear. She limits travel and is no longer willing to go to the mall or into crowds.

Cathy has begun to experience *panic attacks*. Such attacks can be overwhelming, and by definition they sometimes occur out of the blue when there is no reason to become afraid.

Cathy does not understand why she is suddenly feeling this way. During her first episode she thought she was having a heart attack. Like many others, she thought she was dying. After the second attack, Cathy went to the emergency room of her local hospital. They checked her out and reassured her that her heart was fine. But she continued to be afraid about what was really wrong with her.

Very often neither the sufferers of panic attacks nor their doctors recognize panic attacks. Typically a patient may go to as many as seven different doctors before her condition is correctly diagnosed. A medical evaluation is needed to rule out other possible causes of these symptoms. Finding out that the problem is "just" a panic attack, not a heart attack, is a big step toward regaining peace of mind. Many others have experienced this same fright, and it can be controlled.

A panic attack is defined as four or more of the following symptoms that appear abruptly and peak within minutes:

- Pounding heart, or rapid heart rate
- Sweating
- Trembling or shaking
- Sensations of shortness of breath or smothering
- Feeling of choking
- Chest pain or discomfort
- Nausea or abdominal distress
- Feeling dizzy, unsteady, lightheaded, or faint
- Feelings of unreality (*derealization*) or feeling detached from oneself (*depersonalization*)
- Fear of losing control or going crazy
- Fear of dying
- Numbness or tingling sensations
- Chills or hot flushes

The brief duration of panic attack episodes is an important factor in diagnosing panic disorder. True panic attacks do not last for hours or all day. However, the person having the attack often feels shaken and nervous about whether it could happen again.

When someone begins to develop panic attacks, it is not unusual for them to become avoidant. They may stay away from where they were when the attacks began. They may avoid locations where it would be embarrassing or frightening if they had another attack. This avoiding behavior is a secondary problem to the original panic attacks, but may continue even after the panic attacks have been controlled.

When it is extreme, this fearful behavior is called *agoraphobia*, and is a possible complication of panic disorder. People with agoraphobia strongly avoid situations in which they fear having a panic attack. They may especially fear crowds, public transportation, open spaces, enclosed places, being outside the home alone, or any place where they would feel trapped if another attack occurred. They may become so withdrawn that they no longer leave their house. They may be unable to work or attend school and may be highly dependent on others to care for them. They are essentially trapped in their own home by their illness, and they may continue this way for years if there is no effective intervention.

Cathy later was referred to a psychiatrist, who quickly diagnosed her problem. Her psychiatrist started her on a very low dose of an SSRI antidepressant. This medication prevented further attacks. To help overcome her avoidant behavior (she does not go shopping, for example), Cathy also began individual therapy. In time she was able to conquer her fear of crowds and to resume her full range of activities.

SPECIFIC PHOBIA

Mona used to enjoy road trips. Now she is scared to drive on the interstate. A severe car accident three years ago destroyed her confidence in her driving. When she even thinks about driving on the interstate now, her heart starts to race and she feels overwhelmed. She can only visit her elderly mother if she can find someone else to drive her. She hates that her life has been so strongly affected, but she can't find a way to get rid of her fear.

Mona's car accident has led her to develop a phobia, which is a fear of a specific situation or object. In her case the phobia is driving. It is not unusual for people to develop a phobia after a traumatic experience. For example, some acquire a fear of dogs after suffering a dog bite, especially if the bite occurred during childhood. Fear of snakes, elevators, flying, injections, the sight of blood, and heights are other common phobias.

A traumatic event is not a necessary component of a phobia. Family attitudes, parental fears, and cultural expectations can play a role in what someone comes to dread. Media exposure can also influence the development of fears, such as when a young child is subjected to a horror movie. I know of a child exposed to a horror movie who was for years afraid of clowns.

Phobias are the most common psychiatric disorders. If not challenged they can persist for years or even for a lifetime. They may or may not create difficulties in functioning, depending on the nature of the phobia and the person's lifestyle.

Some amount of anxiety is present in all of our lives. You can probably recall situations in which you overcame fears. Do you remember how anxious you felt when you first got behind the wheel of a car, or your first day of school, or your first day at a new job? The difference for someone with a phobia is that their anxiety is more intense and out of proportion to the situation.

Your phobia may not require treatment if you can easily avoid the situations or objects that you fear without any consequence for your relationships or your lifestyle. However, a phobia can be disabling. For example, a fear of elevators may be difficult to ignore for someone who lives in New York City, whereas it might be controllable for a rural resident, at least as long as that person is able-bodied and can manage stairs.

SOCIAL ANXIETY DISORDER (SOCIAL PHOBIA)

Elaine is painfully shy. She is lonely and desperately wants friends, but she is afraid of being judged harshly. She fears disapproval from others and wants to avoid attention. She tries to stay away from group activities.

At work, Elaine tries to keep a "low profile." When she walks down the hall, she avoids eye contact with others. Once a month she is expected to attend a staff meeting, and she is terrified that she will have to speak in front of the group.

Elaine rarely goes to lunch with her co-workers and never goes to parties. She is self-conscious and fears criticism about any comment she might make, how she looks, even what she eats. She feels most comfortable when she is home alone.

Elaine suffers from social anxiety disorder. People who have this disorder look for ways to avoid social situations that cause them so much distress. They realize that their anxiety is excessive but cannot find ways to control their feelings. They fear scrutiny and worry that they will be humiliated, embarrassed, or rejected by others.

Social anxiety can severely limit work performance and the development of relationships. People like Elaine are less likely to be successful at work, get promoted, function academically, and develop intimate relationships. They are less likely to marry. They may seek relief through drinking or illicit drug use (including inappropriate use of addictive anxiety medications). And they may develop depression together with the anxiety.

OBSESSIVE-COMPULSIVE DISORDER

Valerie has a secret. She checks and rechecks her home door locks. She has a ritual every night in which she checks all her doors again and again, sometimes as many as 20 times. She has even driven home from work to make sure that she remembered to lock the doors. She also counts the ceiling tiles at her office. She knows these rituals make no sense and is embarrassed by them, so she does not reveal them to anyone. A few months ago she also started to fear that she might have run over someone in her car while returning from work. This thought terrified her, and now she circles back to that place in the road when she is feeling particularly anxious, to see with her own eyes that no one has been harmed.

Valerie has obsessive-compulsive disorder (OCD). You may be familiar with this disorder due to media, such as the television show *Monk* and the movie *As Good as It Gets*. Valerie is not alone in keeping her obsessions and compulsions a secret. Many who suffer from OCD are aware that their fears are not rational, and they do their best to hide them from others.

OCD includes two parts: *obsessions*, which are unwanted and intrusive thoughts, impulses, or mental images, and *compulsions*, which are behaviors that are performed in response to the thoughts. Obsessions are different from real-life worries and are usually recognized as being unrealistic. They can become troubling and sometimes disturbing.

Common obsessions include:

- Fear of contamination, including dirt or germs
- Doubts (such as worrying whether something has been omitted or an error has occurred)
- Need for order or symmetry
- Recurrent sexual thoughts and images
- Aggressive or frightening impulses

Compulsive behaviors are carried out to reduce the anxiety of the obsessions. Sometimes rituals are developed that must be followed for the person to feel okay. Common compulsions are:

- Repeated washing, such as hand-washing, repeated laundering of clothing, showering
- Counting
- Repeating words silently
- Checking, such as whether the doors are locked or whether some error has occurred at work or while driving
- Putting objects in a certain order

OCD can start during childhood. Typically this condition begins gradually and is hidden by the child for weeks or months to avoid embarrassment. Some children may abruptly exhibit symptoms. Strangely, the onset of the obsessions and compulsions sometimes occurs when a child develops a sore throat. Two decades ago Susan Swedo and her colleagues at the National Institutes of Health identified an association between this abrupt-onset childhood-onset OCD and streptococcal throat infections;

they named the syndrome pediatric autoimmune neuropsychiatric disorder associated with streptococcus (PANDAS). In PANDAS, an autoimmune reaction to strep throat can result in the development of OCD symptoms.

Several variants of OCD have now been identified. *Hoarding disorder* is a recently recognized condition and within *DSM-5* it is classified as being related to OCD. In a hoarding disorder, someone has difficulty discarding or parting with possessions, and thus accumulates things that congest active living space. For these individuals, the hoarding behavior may result in social and occupational problems and significant distress.

Trichotillomania (hair-pulling disorder) is another OCD-related condition that has been defined within *DSM-5*. Women with trichotillomania pull their own hair out repeatedly. They try to stop themselves but are unable to do so, and they may develop patterns of baldness. The most common sites are the scalp, eyebrows, and eyelids, although other sites are possible.

Another newly recognized variant of OCD that is identified in *DSM-5* is *excoriation (skin-picking) disorder.* The essential feature of this disorder is recurrent picking at one's own skin, especially the face, arms, and hands. Picking may be done with the fingernails or with tweezers or other tools. Skin may also be rubbed, squeezed, lanced, or bitten. The majority of individuals with this disorder spend at least an hour a day picking and resisting the urge to pick. This behavior causes significant distress to these individuals and can result in social and occupational impairment.

Body dysmorphic disorder also has been classified as OCD-related in the *DSM-5*. In this disorder, there is a preoccupation with one or more *perceived* defects or flaws in physical appearance that are not observable to other people or that appear slight to other people. These individuals perform repetitive behaviors (such as checking the mirror or excessive grooming) or mental acts (such as comparing themselves with others) in response to their concerns. Their obsessive concern about flaws in their appearance often interferes with their relationships and occupation.

ANXIOUS DEPRESSION

Sophie started feeling anxious at the same time that she became depressed. Her marriage is crumbling, she was recently diagnosed with cancer, and she feels totally alone in the world. She was previously a calm person, but now finds she is overcome with fears.

Sophie displays a common pattern, the coexisting presence of anxious symptoms with depression. We might think of depression and anxiety as being flip sides of the same coin. The feelings are often mixed and occur together. In the past we thought that they required different types of treatments, but fortunately we have approaches now that will work for both anxiety and depression simultaneously. We will discuss those treatments later in this chapter.

POSTTRAUMATIC STRESS DISORDER

Julie was returning from a study session on campus when a man grabbed her from behind and brutally raped her. She was terrified and devastated. The rapist has not been found, and she lives in fear that he might come back. She finds herself suddenly reliving the attack. She has nightmares about it often and wakes up screaming. She is very jumpy now, easily startled. It is hard for her to trust men, even her long-time male friends.

Julie's life truly was in danger on the day she was raped. She felt lucky to survive. The fear that now haunts her began on the day of that attack. Her anxiety began with a real threat to her safety. Sadly, the fear that was born on that day continues to rob her life of its fullness.

Those who suffer from posttraumatic stress disorder (PTSD) have experienced an extreme trauma, in many cases a trauma in which their life was in danger. Afterwards, they cannot escape the horror. They may experience one or more of these symptoms:

- Repeated disturbing memories of the event
- Repeated nightmares about the event
- Flashbacks, in which they feel as if the trauma were recurring
- Intense distress when exposed to cues that represent the event
- Physical reactivity, such as shaking or other nervousness, when reminded of the event

In addition to experiencing these symptoms, people with PTSD often become avoidant and numb, with feelings such as:

- Emotional numbing (feeling as though they don't care about anything)
- Detachment (from feelings and from others)
- Amnesia (being unable to remember important parts of the trauma)
- Greatly reduced desire to participate in significant activities
- Reduced range of emotions (such as not being able to have loving feelings)
- Sense of foreshortened future (such as no longer expecting a normal life span)

An additional component of PTSD is feeling overly reactive and aroused, as shown by the following:

- Sleep problems (difficulty falling or staying asleep)
- Irritability or outbursts of anger
- Concentration (difficulty concentrating)
- Hyper-vigilance (feeling always on watch)
- Startling easily

PTSD is one of the most disabling forms of anxiety disorder. It often is associated with depression and lowered self-esteem. The emotions triggered by the traumatic event may be hard ever to escape. People who were sexually molested may develop PTSD and feel consumed by anger toward the person who abused them and others who failed to protect them. Others may develop PTSD after a car accident, for example, or another situation that does not involve a specific abuser. PTSD is also well known to occur after military and combat experiences. Many people with PTSD turn to alcohol or drugs or become sexually promiscuous. They may feel that sex is the only way to feel validated, and yet sex does not bring the comfort they seek. Some people with PTSD engage in other self-destructive behaviors such as cutting themselves. They may feel worthless and develop thoughts of killing themselves.

What Can You Do If You Have Anxiety?

If you can identify with any of the anxiety disorders described in this chapter, know that there is help for you. Recovery is not simple and it may require a lot of effort on your part, but you can get better.

The approach you take depends on the type of anxiety you are experiencing. I will discuss both general strategies that can help anyone who suffers from anxious feelings, as well as treatments for more severe anxiety and for specific disorders.

USE RELAXATION TECHNIQUES

Relaxation is a state that you can learn and practice. There are several techniques that may help you.

- Abdominal breathing. When our bodies feel anxious, our breathing becomes more rapid and shallow. Our heart rate increases and we perspire more. When you feel anxious, breathe deeply and slowly. Simply taking a step back from your thoughts and feelings, focusing on your breathing, can in itself be soothing. We can teach our bodies to be calmer by starting with our breathing. This type of slow breathing will send a message to your brain and body to calm down. Various ways of breathing can calm. Consciously choosing to breathe deeply from the abdomen serves to restore calm. To practice abdominal breathing, slowly inhale through your nose, counting to four as you do. Hold the air for a count of seven. Exhale through your mouth while counting to eight, contracting your abdominal muscles to expel all the air.

• Progressive muscle relaxation. This approach involves slowly tensing and then relaxing the muscles of each region of the body. Start by tensing the muscles in your toes for at least five seconds and then relaxing them for 15 seconds. Repeat the process. Slowly work your way up the body to your head and neck area. Pay special attention to your physical sensations.

• Visual imagery. You simply close your eyes and envision the most beautiful, restful, idyllic setting that you can imagine. This may be a place that you have visited, a special spot in your life, or it could be imaginary. It could be the beach or the mountains or a field full of flowers. Allow yourself to experience the sensations of this setting. Feel the sunshine, smell the ocean, sense the breezes. Cultivate this imagery so you can easily return to it when you have a few minutes to take a break during an otherwise stressful day.

• Music. Listening to music is another way to unwind. Spend some time on your music collection and identify artists and songs that soothe you. Listening carefully to music is not only pleasant, it fills your mind so your body will naturally relax.

• Massage. If you have not had one, you may find a new way of relaxing by having a professional therapeutic massage. Or you could ask a friend to give you one. The physical release may do wonders to help you feel more at ease.

• Biofeedback. This refers to the process of learning relaxation using physiologic measures that give you "feedback" on your state of activity. A variety of devices can be used to inform you when you are making healthy changes in your heart rate, brain waves, skin conductance, and other measures of your body's activity level. Over time you can learn to relax using such methods.

EXERCISE

Exercise has the remarkable ability to shift your mood and relieve your anxiety. If you can manage a walk outdoors, you will also get the additional benefit of time to reflect and enjoy the beauty of nature, and a dose of sunshine. Take time to notice the little things. You may want to walk with a friend, or listen to music you enjoy, or simply savor the time for yourself. Meeting a personal goal to walk at least several times a week may do wonders to reduce your anxiety level. There is evidence that resistance exercise (weight lifting) may also have benefit for anxiety.

MAKE NUTRITIONAL CHANGES

- Eat healthy meals. Your diet has a big influence on how you feel, and when chosen carefully, can help you feel calmer. Your goal is to eat well-balanced meals and avoid allowing yourself to become too hungry. Learn to eat several smaller meals a day, with an emphasis on proteins and complex carbohydrates such as whole-grain breads, pasta, starchy vegetables, and beans. Such a diet can help to keep your blood sugar and your mood more stable. It is especially helpful to eat a breakfast that includes protein.
- Reduce caffeine. Anyone with an anxiety problem should reduce or eliminate caffeine use, since it can cause anxiety, and for some it can also trigger panic attacks or cause insomnia.
- Limit sugar. A diet high in sugar also promotes more anxiety. It is common for those who eat something with a high sugar content to feel nervous about an hour or two after eating it. The body releases insulin after you eat a simple sugar, and the insulin causes your blood sugar to drop lower than it was before you ate. Low blood sugar

may cause you to feel shaky and uneasy. In contrast, complex carbohydrates such as whole grains help to increase the level of serotonin in your brain, which has a calming effect.

- Stay hydrated. Drink plenty of water throughout the day. The amount you should consume depends on your age, diet, and level of physical activity, but aiming for the traditional eight 8-ounce glasses of fluids per day is a good place to start (all fluids you drink count). If you become dehydrated, you are likely to feel weak and shaky.
- Limit your alcohol use. Small amounts of alcohol have been touted for their health benefits, but if you drink excessively you are likely to feel more anxious. In addition, excessive alcohol can interfere with sleep.

PRACTICE GOOD SLEEP HYGIENE

Poor sleep is often a symptom of anxiety disorders. There are several strategies that can help you to sleep. Establish a regular routine at bedtime that is calming, and follow the recommendations previously described in chapter 6. See table 1 in that chapter for a list of medications that may be prescribed for you to aid with sleep, but be cautious since many of these medications are meant for short-term use only. Strive to develop healthy habits and avoid physical or psychological dependence on sleep agents.

PERFORM MEDITATION AND YOGA

In recent years, both meditation and yoga have become popular as methods for soothing nerves. The many meditation techniques all share the central quality of promoting calmness and mindfulness. Some types of meditation are associated with religious and spiritual practices, but many types are not.

Some meditation techniques encourage you to focus your breath, while others center on your thought process. Some techniques teach you to concentrate on a single word or image. Another technique teaches you to observe, but not react to, your experiences from moment to moment, without trying to control the focus.

Numerous studies have shown there are many physical benefits from meditating. For people who regularly practice meditation, blood pressure is lowered, pulse is slowed, and even the galvanic skin response (a measure of anxiety) is reduced. Emotional benefits are more difficult to prove, but many practitioners of meditation report feeling calmer and more focused. Meditation has been used for pain control and treating depression, as well as stress reduction.

Yoga is a collection of techniques that also may be associated with spiritual goals. For many, it is a physical exercise regimen that helps to improve balance and gain serenity. For some, yoga is a means toward enlightenment.

Yoga originally developed in Asia, but now many Westerners practice both meditation and yoga. Yoga is so common that many exercise centers now offer classes in it.

INVESTIGATE HERBAL AND VITAMIN SUPPLEMENTS

A variety of herbal and vitamin treatments are touted as beneficial for stress these days, but many lack any evidence of effectiveness. I urge caution in using treatments that are not approved by the FDA since the production of these supplements may not be carefully monitored. That means that there is uncertainty about their exact content and safety. Dietary and herbal supplements may contain impurities, such as lead and arsenic, and may cause adverse effects and drug interactions. Be sure to tell your doctor about any vitamins or supplements that you are taking because they might react negatively with prescribed medication.

PRAY

Every faith has prayers that encourage you to look outside yourself and find hope and peace. When you are feeling anxious, you may find it difficult to pray. Try not to blame yourself for feeling anxiety. Anxiety is not a reflection of your lack of faith, but your faith may help you to become calmer. It may be helpful to meet with your minister, priest, rabbi, or other spiritual advisor, or to look at books about your faith to find specific prayers that promote wellness. You may also benefit by joining a prayer group or other small group through your religious affiliation. You may find that praying with others helps you to have more hope and also gives you a larger sense of perspective as you hear the concerns of others.

CONSIDER COGNITIVE BEHAVIORAL THERAPY

Automatic thoughts can promote anxiety, just as thoughts can lead to or increase depression. The same cognitive therapy techniques that were discussed in chapter 6 for depression can also be used to help overcome anxiety. For example, someone who becomes nervous at the thought of giving a speech can learn to identify specific thoughts that promote more anxiety (for example, *What if I forget what I am saying? What if someone asks me a question that I don't know how to answer?*). If you analyze the thought process that leads to more anxious feelings, you are better able to introduce alternative thoughts that are more calming (*I will have prompts with me in case I forget. I can ask the person with the question what they think, or I could admit that I don't know the answer and then offer to find out*).

One example of an automatic thought that promotes more anxiety is called *catastrophizing*. You worry that if a certain negative event were to occur, it would be a catastrophe that you could not handle. Such thoughts increase your fears and panic, even if the event never happens. Thinking that you could not handle a situation also is demoralizing, and can create a spiral of anxiety that feeds on itself.

Cognitive therapy helps you feel alternative, more soothing thoughts. In the case of catastrophizing, for example, you may benefit from recalling the other challenges that you have successfully met. You are likely stronger than you think you are, and there are many affirming thoughts that may help you realize this.

Shifting your focus to more positive, hopeful thoughts can help you to be calmer and more confident.

TRY OTHER THERAPIES

Exposure therapy. This behavioral approach is especially helpful for treating people who have phobias and/or OCD. It assumes that if a person avoids an object that is feared, the object will continue to seem frightful. On the other hand, if you push yourself to confront the very object or situation that you fear, over time you will find that the fear fades away. That is, you will become *desensitized* to the object. This approach requires courage because it compels you to face your fears directly. The key is to find a way to push yourself to do the very thing that you are afraid of, and eventually it will seem less frightening.

An example can illustrate this technique. Suppose you are afraid of elevators. If you always take the stairs to avoid elevators then your fear of elevators will probably continue. Exposure therapy helps you confront your fear. You might start by envisioning yourself riding an elevator. If your phobia is severe, the very thought of such a ride might cause you to feel nervous. Nevertheless, over time you would probably get accustomed to the idea of yourself in an elevator without feeling so anxious. Next, you might stand by an elevator and watch other people enter and exit. You might ask someone to ride with you for one floor and then get off. Once you felt comfortable, you could ride the elevator by yourself for one floor. Eventually you would ride up and down many floors unaccompanied. Each time you pushed yourself a little harder, your anxiety would temporarily increase. But both your body and your emotions would adjust, so that over time you would be able to do each step with less anxiety. Your heart would no longer race at the thought of elevators. You would be able to accomplish your goal of overcoming your fear if you did it slowly and pushed yourself past the fear.

Obsessive-compulsive disorder is another anxiety disorder that can be treated with a variation of exposure therapy called *exposure and response prevention*, which is designed to prevent the person from the compulsive behavior that typically follows the obsessive thought. Over time, if you continue to be exposed to the fearful situation or thought and are not able to respond with the compulsion, you will find that you are less afraid.

Again, an example may help to clarify this approach. Suppose you are afraid of contamination. You may obsess about cleanliness and feel the need to wash your hands repeatedly after you have somehow contaminated them. Touching a doorknob is a classic example of an action that may elicit the compulsion to wash hands in someone with this form of OCD. To treat this compulsion, you would be encouraged to touch a doorknob and then you would be blocked, or you would block yourself, from your usual hand-washing ritual.

Compulsive behaviors serve to relieve the anxiety generated by obsessive thoughts. If you are prevented from your compulsion, you will likely feel more anxious initially. Over time, your anxiety will diminish and eventually you will no longer require the ritual to feel okay.

Eye Movement Desensitization and Reprocessing (EMDR). In 1989 the psychologist Francine Shapiro created a novel therapy approach for PTSD. EMDR combines several different techniques, including an eye movement exercise. Since it was initially developed, EMDR has been shown to be effective in research studies, but there has been controversy about the role of the eye movements. Some have questioned whether the eye movement component is essential to the method. Nevertheless, EMDR therapy has been endorsed by many professional organizations, and it is widely used for victims of trauma such as military veterans and rape victims.

EMDR weaves together components from several different psychotherapeutic approaches. Treatment moves through phases, with the goal to teach the brain to process experiences differently. The patient reviews initial trauma and current triggers to identify the associated thoughts and feelings. Later, the patient develops healthier images, thoughts, and feelings. Ultimately, the brain learns to react in a healthier way so that the damaging effects from trauma go away. To practice the EMDR technique, a therapist must undergo special training. If you are interested in this treatment, look for a therapist who has been trained to practice EMDR on patients.

Prolonged exposure (PE). In 1984 the psychologist Edna Foa created a specialized therapy approach for PTSD. It is based on cognitive-behavioral principles. Since it was developed, studies have shown it to be highly effective for treating PTSD. This approach incorporates education about common reactions to trauma, using one's imagination to relive memories of the trauma, and a process to gradually desensitize the patient to the trauma (analogous to the process used to treat phobias). The treatment includes breathing retraining and talking through the trauma. Clinicians throughout the United States and elsewhere have used PE to treat survivors of a variety of traumas.

SEEK AN EVALUATION FOR MEDICATION

For several decades, psychiatrists treated anxiety with anti-anxiety (also called *anxiolytic*) medication and treated depression with antidepressants. Now we know that antidepressant medications can treat both depression and anxiety, and they have the advantage of being nonaddictive (unlike many of the anxiety medications that are prescribed). This recognition has significantly improved treatment of anxiety disorders, but it requires patience for the antidepressant to take effect. The psychiatrist should start with low dosages of antidepressants, since women with anxiety may be especially sensitive to side effects.

The Food and Drug Administration (FDA) has approved many antidepressants to treat specific anxiety disorders (see table 4). Often a medication is created to treat one condition (such as depression) and is later found to be effective for other conditions. It is intriguing to discover that medications can treat a variety of disorders. Physicians are allowed to prescribe medications for indications that the FDA has not approved (so-called off-label uses), but drug companies are not allowed to market these medications for specific disorders until the FDA approves use of the medication for that purpose. Many SSRIs are prescribed for off-label uses.

TABLE 4   *Antidepressants Approved for Treating Anxiety by the Food and Drug Administration (FDA)*

Condition	Drugs approved by FDA for use
SELECTIVE SEROTONIN REUPTAKE INHIBITORS (SSRIs)	
Obsessive-compulsive disorder (OCD)	Prozac (fluoxetine) Luvox (fluvoxamine) Paxil (paroxetine) Zoloft (sertraline)
Panic disorder	Prozac (fluoxetine) Paxil (paroxetine) Zoloft (sertraline)
Social anxiety disorder	Paxil (paroxetine) Zoloft (sertraline)
Generalized anxiety disorder (GAD)	Lexapro (escitalopram) Paxil (paroxetine)
Posttraumatic Stress Disorder (PTSD)	Paxil (paroxetine) Zoloft (sertraline)
SEROTONIN NOREPINEPHRINE REUPTAKE INHIBITORS (SNRIs)	
Generalized anxiety disorder (GAD)	Effexor (venlafaxine) Cymbalta (duloxetine)
Social anxiety disorder Panic disorder	Effexor (venlafaxine)
TRICYCLIC ANTIDEPRESSANTS	
Obsessive-compulsive disorder (OCD)	Anafranil (clomipramine)

SSRIs are used to treat anxiety disorders. The FDA approved the following SSRIs to treat OCD: Prozac (fluoxetine), Luvox (fluvoxamine), Paxil (paroxetine), and Zoloft (sertraline). The FDA approved Prozac (fluoxetine), Paxil (paroxetine), and Zoloft (sertraline) to treat panic disorder; Paxil (paroxetine) and Zoloft (sertraline) to treat social anxiety disorder; Paxil (paroxetine) and Lexapro (escitalopram) to treat generalized anxiety disorder (GAD); and Paxil (paroxetine) and Zoloft (sertraline) to treat

TABLE 5   *Nonaddicting Anxiety Medications*

Brand name	Generic name	Recommended dose range*
Buspar	buspirone	20–30 mg/day taken in divided doses
Vistaril, Atarax, Marax	hydroxyzine	50–100 mg/day in divided doses

*As of 2015.

posttraumatic stress disorder (PTSD). Over time, it is common for the FDA to approve additional indications for medications if there is convincing evidence that the drug works for other disorders.

The tricyclic antidepressant Anafranil (clomipramine) was the first drug approved by the FDA for treating OCD.

The serotonin norepinephrine reuptake inhibitors (SNRIs) may also be of benefit for the anxiety disorders. Effexor (venlafaxine) and Cymbalta (duloxetine) are FDA-approved for treating GAD. Effexor (venlafaxine) is also approved by the FDA for treating social anxiety disorder and panic disorder.

Several anxiety medications are available that have the advantage of being non-addicting. Buspar (buspirone) is FDA-approved for GAD. Its side effects are mild for most people, primarily slight sedation. It does not work immediately, but within a couple of weeks it may produce a calming effect. Vistaril (hydroxyzine) is another non-addicting medication that is sometimes prescribed for anxiety. The side effects of these two medications include sedation and they can be taken at bedtime to improve sleep. They can also be taken during the day, but as with any other sedating medication, be cautious about activities such as driving if you feel overly sedated and report this to your doctor.

Benzodiazepines are an older family of anxiety medications, and they are still frequently used today (see table 6). However, they have the big drawback of being highly addictive. They provide quick relief from anxious feelings but may also lead to more anx-

TABLE 6 *Benzodiazepine Medications*

Brand name	Generic name	Recommended dose range*
Ativan	lorazepam	2–6† mg/day in divided doses
Dalmane	flurazepam	15–30† mg at bedtime
Klonopin	clonazepam	0.5–4† mg/day in divided doses
Librium	chlordiazepoxide	15–40† mg/day in divided doses
Restoril	temazepam	7.5–30† mg/day at bedtime
Serax	oxazepam	30–60† mg/day in divided doses
Tranxene	clorazepate	15–60† mg/day in divided doses
Valium	diazepam	4–40† mg/day in divided doses
Xanax, Xanax XR	alprazolam	0.75–4† mg/day in divided doses

*As of 2015.
†The upper dosages for these drugs are a function of the underlying condition, how long they have been used, and the sensitivity and tolerance of the patient. Beware of taking these medications at the upper limit of the dose range or in combination with other drugs or alcohol, since they may be dangerous.

iety once their effect wears off. I steer my patients away from this family of medications due to the risk of addiction, but many patients are already dependent on them. If someone takes one of these medications for a while, they will become addicted, and then if they do not have that medication, they will experience even more anxiety as a withdrawal symptom. Those who do take benzodiazepines should use the lowest possible dose and never combine them with alcohol, since that can be very dangerous.

In my practice, I use benzodiazepines to prevent patients with panic disorder from developing avoiding behaviors. I will often prescribe a very small quantity of one of these medications and advise my patients to keep it in their purse so they know that if they do have a panic attack, they can "nip it in the bud." This gives them security to go into any situation and get relief if a panic attack should occur.

All benzodiazepines can be addictive. Over time your body can become dependent on this type of medication. You may require higher doses to get the same relief. If you abruptly stop the medication, you will experience withdrawal symptoms, such as anxiety, irritability, and insomnia. This is the problem with this family of medications: they wind up creating the same symptom that they treat, namely, anxiety.

For anyone who becomes dependent on one of the benzodiazepine medications listed here, discontinuation of this medication must be done very slowly. You should prepare yourself for some unpleasant feelings as you withdraw from the medication. Your increase in anxiety will be temporary, and with a gradual approach you will be able to stop your use. In some cases seizures or death can result from withdrawal. If your withdrawal symptoms are severe, your doctor should carefully monitor and manage the withdrawal process. In some instances, this can be done in a hospital setting so that you can be more closely watched.

•

This chapter provides an overview of the various types of anxiety that can occur and various ways to treat them and provide a recipe for peace. As with depression, usually the best way to treat anxiety disorders combines several approaches. There are many ways to learn to overcome your fears. Being trained to think differently and to nurture yourself can be straightforward keys to your happiness. Lifestyle changes and therapy are the best way to begin. If medication is needed, SSRI medications are a good choice. Beware of the "quick fix" of benzodiazepine medications. It is much healthier to use other approaches or medications that can be effective without the risk of long-term addiction.

Therapy is an incredibly effective treatment for anxiety. Regardless of the specific form of therapy, a strong alliance with your therapist can help you to acquire emotional stability. Unfortunately, many people who have anxiety lack a basic sense of security. They may have been damaged in their childhood by abuse, or have had other experiences that cause them to be fearful of the world and of other people. They may be reluctant to engage in therapy, afraid to trust someone with their innermost thoughts and feelings. They may doubt whether it will really help. They may think that the process will stir up their anxieties and cause them to feel worse. They may question whether the value of therapy is worth the cost. Since therapy is a very personal experience, these reservations are understandable. However, many, many women have told me how much therapy has helped them. Therapy can save your life. If you find the right therapist whom you can trust and with whom you can feel a connection, you can learn to feel safer in the world and overcome your fears.

RECOMMENDED RESOURCES

Edmund J. Bourne, Ph D. *The Anxiety and Phobia Workbook,* 4th edition. Oakland, CA: New Harbinger Publications, 2005.

Michelle G. Craske, PhD, and Holly Hazlett-Stevens, PhD. *Women Who Worry Too Much: How to Stop Worry and Anxiety from Ruining Relationships, Work and Fun.* Oakland, CA: New Harbinger Publications, 2005.

David V. Sheehan, MD. *The Anxiety Disease: New Hope for the Millions Who Suffer From Anxiety.* New York: Bantam Books, 1983.

Claire Weekes, MD. *Hope and Help for Your Nerves.* New York: Penguin Group, 1969.

Margaret Wehrenberg, PsyD. *The 10 Best-Ever Anxiety Management Techniques: Understanding How Your Brain Makes You Anxious and What You Can Do to Change It.* New York: W.W. Norton, 2008.

CHAPTER 8

Women and Substance Abuse

Eva's husband said that she was no longer the woman he married and that she had to get some help for her drinking problem if she wanted to save their marriage.

Eva works full time as a medical office manager and finds the job demanding and stressful. There are always problems to solve and difficult people to please. She feels caught in the middle, with much responsibility but little authority. She is the mother of two school-age children. One of them has ADHD and is difficult to parent. She and her husband have been having a lot of arguments lately about child rearing.

Eva started drinking during college and drank "socially" for several years. In the last few years, her drinking increased as her stress level increased. She prefers wine and drinks several glasses every night. On the weekends she sometimes drinks an entire bottle. Sometimes she feels shaky in the mornings and wants a drink. She thinks she is neglecting her children and she feels guilty, but it seems the only time she feels good is after a drink or two. One evening last month she drove after drinking and worried that if she got pulled over she would get a DUI. She can see that she is starting to put herself and her family in danger, but she does not see herself as an "alcoholic." She resents that her husband thinks she needs help. She thinks she could stop on her own, but in the last several years the longest she has gone without a drink is one day.

How Does Substance Abuse Affect Women?

Eva has developed a reliance on alcohol, so it will be hard for her to stop. Her drinking is starting to cause problems for her. Her body and her emotions have become "dependent." She is starting to show signs of withdrawal, like the "shakes," when she does not have a drink.

Women are less likely to develop alcohol problems than men. But once they do begin to drink, they tend to become addicted more rapidly and to have more physical health problems such as cirrhosis of the liver, cardiomyopathy (heart disease), and problems in thinking. Women drinkers also have higher rates of breast cancer, hypertension, and stroke.

Illegal drug abuse has similar gender differences. Women are less likely than men to abuse drugs such as marijuana, cocaine, and narcotics as well as prescription drugs. However, once they do begin to abuse these drugs, they more rapidly become addicted and develop serious problems from their drug use. They may combine the drugs that they use. They also often drink and use drugs. These combinations carry additional risks. Drug use may affect their relationships, health, and employment, as well as create the potential for legal problems.

There are unique issues around alcohol or drug addictions in women, such as the impact of alcohol and drugs during pregnancy. Substance abuse during pregnancy can be harmful to the mother's ability to support her own pregnancy and can damage the prenatal development of her baby. During pregnancy, virtually any substance abuse by the mother poses a danger to both mother and fetus. Drinking alcohol can cause the child lifelong physical and behavioral problems, including fetal alcohol syndrome. Babies with this syndrome may be born with mental retardation, experience slow growth, and have other physical abnormalities including possible heart defects. Narcotic drugs, such as Lortab and Oxycontin, can cause withdrawal symptoms in the baby. Benzodiazepines, such as Valium and Xanax, can also cause withdrawal symptoms in the baby, and there is a greater risk of birth defects such as cleft lip. Use of other illicit drugs during pregnancy can affect the baby as well.

Women can also be affected by substance abuse if they have a spouse, child, or other family member who is addicted. Many women find themselves in such a situation, and they can feel consumed by the problem of substance abuse in their loved one. They find themselves taking care of the addicted family member, cleaning up after them, covering up for them when work or social problems develop. The addicted family member may be emotionally or physically abusing them. They often sacrifice their own needs in order to take care of the addicted family member.

Codependency is a term that was originally created to describe the characteristics of spouses of alcoholics, but it has now been popularized and extended to describe more broadly the psychological phenomenon that can develop in family and friends in response to an addiction. When a woman is codependent, she focuses her energy on taking care of someone else, even when she is being controlled and manipulated. Many women and men with addictions are maintained by the support of codependent family members and friends. It is helpful for all involved to understand these concepts so the patterns can be broken.

Why Do Some Women Become Addicted to Alcohol or Drugs?

Addiction has many causes. One risk factor for developing alcohol problems is a family history of alcoholism. There is a genetic component to this disorder. Furthermore, growing up where alcohol or drugs are used increases the likelihood that a girl may later abuse substances herself. She may learn to turn to alcohol or drugs when stressed.

Another risk factor for substance abuse is a history of sexual abuse or sexual assault. The rate of substance abuse in women who were sexually abused is three to four times higher than the rate for women who have not been abused.

Drugs that doctors prescribe to treat anxiety and pain can be addicting. Women experience anxiety disorders more often than men, and many are prescribed benzodiazepine medications, such as Xanax (alprazolam). As discussed in chapter 7, some of the anti-anxiety medications can lead to dependence, especially short-acting medications such as alprazolam. Some women also develop a "tolerance" and start taking larger amounts of the medication to get the same effect. While benzodiazepines can help women with anxiety, they should be used very cautiously. Similarly, narcotic medications for pain can be beneficial when taken as prescribed but should be used with care to avoid addiction.

Substance Abuse and Depression

Women who have depression may abuse alcohol and drugs to relieve their emotional distress. It is often hard to know which came first—depression or substance abuse—and whether one problem led to the other. Women with depression may be trying to "self-medicate" with alcohol or drugs. For example, they may think that they will feel better if they drink a little, and sometimes they do feel better for a short time. However, over time their drinking tends to make their depression worse. It also makes it more difficult for depression treatments to be effective.

The other scenario would be for alcohol or drug abuse to precede the development of depression. Alcohol and drug problems tend to be self-destructive over time. It is common for those who suffer from these problems to have deteriorating lives and lifestyles. They may lose relationships, jobs, money, and support from others as they progress with their substance abuse. Commonly, depression follows these losses.

"Dual diagnosis" is the term used to describe the association of substance abuse and mental illness. Roughly 30 percent of individuals with mental illness also abuse alcohol or drugs, and 60 percent of people who have bipolar disorder also have a substance abuse disorder. Ideally, these problems would be treated together. Usually the substance abuse is treated first, since it is difficult to effectively treat depression while someone is actively drinking or using drugs.

What Can You Do If You Think You or Someone You Care About May Be Abusing Alcohol and Drugs?

OVERCOME DENIAL

Denial is the first hurdle to overcome in addressing alcohol and drug abuse. A woman who is abusing alcohol or drugs may not be able to admit that she has a problem. Family members and friends may confront her together in what is called an "intervention," to help her see that she has a problem and guide her toward getting help. It is wise to carefully plan and prepare for such an intervention, collect evidence about the problems that have been observed by others, and develop a specific plan for getting into treatment. Professional substance abuse counselors or other mental health professionals can help the family make these plans and can attend the intervention if the family wants them and finds it appropriate.

UNDERGO DETOXIFICATION

Detoxification ("detox") is frequently needed to manage withdrawal symptoms at the beginning of treatment. This first step consists of safely discontinuing use of the alcohol and/or drugs. Use should be slowly decreased and then stopped. During this process, many people have withdrawal symptoms, such as shakiness, anxiety, clammy skin, nausea, rapid heart rate, and sweating, especially if use is stopped abruptly. Ideally, stopping the use gradually minimizes withdrawal symptoms. Detoxification can be done either in a hospital or at an outpatient clinic setting and requires approximately five to seven days. During this treatment, medication can help reduce withdrawal symptoms and prevent serious problems such as seizures or delirium tremens ("DTs"), a potentially life-threatening syndrome. DT symptoms can include confusion, agitation, hallucinations, fever, high blood pressure, and fast heart rate. DTs are uncommon and can be prevented with an adequate detox program. Overall, the withdrawal process from alcohol and other drugs is unpleasant, and I often tell patients to keep those feelings in mind so they won't relapse and have to go through it again. Drug and alcohol rehabilitation can start during detox, with a focus on relapse prevention.

PARTICIPATE IN REHABILITATION

The next step is a rehabilitation program, if available, to prevent recurrence of the substance abuse, accompanied by treatment for the depression. Longer-term rehabilitation programs often use the "twelve-step" approach. The twelve-step philosophy requires total abstinence from alcohol and drugs to achieve and maintain sobriety. This approach uses a number of concepts and behaviors, including turning your life over to a higher power, being honest, and finding a way to make amends to those who have been wronged because of your addiction.

Alcoholics Anonymous (AA) and Narcotics Anonymous (NA) are free self-help groups with chapters across the country. These groups also use the twelve-step approach. Support from a group can be critical in helping to avoid a relapse. Groups can be especially useful for women, since a group can provide connection with others with the common goal of sobriety. Many communities have "women's meetings," in which it may be easier for women with substance abuse to support one another than it would be in a mixed-sex setting.

For family members, Al-Anon and Alateen are free self-help groups that can provide needed support. In these confidential meetings, family members can help each other learn to recognize their own patterns of behavior and can increase their understanding of the disease process of addiction.

GET EVALUATED FOR MEDICATIONS

Women who abuse substances and who have major depression or posttraumatic stress disorder need to get treatment for both conditions. These disorders may require psychotherapy and/ or medications as discussed in previous chapters.

Medications are sometimes prescribed after detoxification to reduce the risk of relapse. Antabuse (disulfiram) may be given as part of treatment for problem drinking, and causes a very unpleasant and potentially dangerous reaction if you drink. Vivitrol (naltrexone) and Campral (acamprosate) are also sometimes given to reduce cravings for alcohol and the risk of relapse.

Narcotic addiction can be treated with methadone and buprenorphine, two synthetic narcotics that lack the euphoric effects seen with other narcotics and have less potential for abuse. They are used both temporarily and also for long-term maintenance. There has been controversy around their use, but evidence suggests that prescribing these agents is the safest way to manage narcotic addiction. These agents prevent withdrawal from opiates such as Lortab (acetaminophen and hydrocodone), Oxycontin (oxycodone), and heroin. Typically, methadone treatment requires that the person go to a specialized clinic daily. There are significant risks if methadone is taken with other narcotic drugs. Buprenorphine is a newer opiate substitute that can be obtained at the office of a doctor who is trained and certified to prescribe it. Subutex is the marketed version of buprenorphine alone, while Suboxone refers to the combination of buprenorphine and naloxone (a drug that blocks the effects of narcotics) that was created to prevent abuse. Both methadone and buprenorphine allow someone with an addiction to narcotics to continue to function.

Women who are pregnant and addicted to narcotics (heroin, morphine, Oxycontin, Lortab, or others) need help for themselves as well as protection for their unborn babies. Both methadone and buprenorphine have been used during pregnancy and have been demonstrated to be safer than continued narcotic abuse. They reduce the risk of infectious diseases such as hepatitis and HIV and other risks during pregnancy that may occur if the mother is still abusing opiates. However, these medications enter the fetal bloodstream through the placenta. At birth these babies experience withdrawal, known as the neonatal abstinence syndrome (NAS). The symptoms of NAS include irritability, tremors, vomiting, difficulty breathing, poor sleep, and low-grade fevers. Many newborns with NAS require hospitalization in neonatal intensive care units. A recent study compared the effectiveness of methadone versus buprenorphine during pregnancy and found that infants whose mothers were treated with buprenorphine had milder withdrawal symptoms and were able to recover more quickly than those treated with methadone. The use of buprenorphine or methadone during pregnancy is recommended for narcotic-addicted women by the American College of Obstetricians and Gynecologists to avoid the greater harm that could occur if the mother returned to using more dangerous street drugs.

SEEK SUPPORT

Women who seek a new, sober life will need support from family and friends who also value sobriety. It may be necessary to seek "different places and different faces" (a recovery slogan) to avoid the pull back into addiction. In other words, women may benefit from avoiding the situations and friends associated with their previous lifestyle and replacing them with healthier activities and friendships (such as hobbies, sports, clubs, or faith-based groups).

Relapse prevention includes learning how to cope with life stresses without turning to the false solution of alcohol or drugs. It helps to develop practical plans, and practice different coping skills, to manage stresses and difficult emotions. Taking a walk, listening to soothing music, writing in a journal, and talking to a friend are just a few of the strategies that may help when times get tough.

AA and NA use sponsors, people who have experienced similar struggles and have learned to maintain their own sobriety. The person with the addiction can talk to and turn to her sponsor when she needs support during her recovery. Sponsors can share strategies that they themselves found helpful and are available if the other person is tempted to relapse. If one sponsor is a not good fit, it's best to find another sponsor—even if it takes two or three tries.

•

Substance abuse in yourself or your family can be destructive, but it can be overcome. Alcohol and drugs are sad substitutes for a sense of balance in life. If you realize you need help, start to change by confiding in someone. Check out the free support groups (as described in this chapter) in your area. You can regain your life and preserve your relationships, and there are many people who will help you.

RECOMMENDED RESOURCES

BOOKS

Anonymous. *Alcoholics Anonymous: The Big Book*, 4th edition (2001). New York: Alcoholics Anonymous World Services, 2001.

Melody Beattie. *Codependent No More: How to Stop Controlling Others and Start Caring for Yourself.* Center City, MN: Hazelden, 1986.

Stephanie S. Covington, PhD. *A Woman's Way through the Twelve Steps.* Center City, MN: Hazelden, 1994.

Lisa M. Najavits, PhD. *A Woman's Addiction Workbook: Your Guide to In-Depth Healing.* Oakland, CA: New Harbinger Publications, 2002.

WEBSITES

For Alcoholics Anonymous self-help groups: www.aa.org

For Narcotics Anonymous self-help groups that include focus on drugs as well as alcohol: www.na.org

For Al-Anon and Al-Ateen self-help groups: http://www.al-anon.alateen.org

CHAPTER 9

Bipolar Disorder in Women

Natalie first came to see me because she was so depressed that she was having trouble with her job and with her family. She felt overwhelmed and unable to focus. She was easily angered by her husband and children and had been yelling at her kids recently. She cried heavily at our first appointment as she told me how down she was feeling. She was having trouble sleeping, had little appetite, and was feeling hopeless. At times suicidal thoughts were coming into her head. Her primary care physician had recently prescribed an antidepressant for her, but so far she was feeling worse and more agitated.

Natalie and I reviewed her history, and she shared with me that several times in her life she had felt unusually energetic. She loved that feeling. She felt on top of the world, very confident, and able to do anything she tried. During those periods, she had so much energy that she barely needed to sleep at night. She would accomplish much more than usual and feel great about herself. She knew that at times she annoyed other people because she talked so fast they couldn't get a word in edgewise. She also got herself in trouble at those times by going on spending sprees that she couldn't afford. These periods typically lasted about a week.

Natalie has come to fear her emotional roller coaster of feeling very "up" and then very "down." Although she enjoyed her periods of feeling "up," she was beginning to realize they are not good for her.

What Is Bipolar Disorder?

Natalie's history is not unusual for someone who has bipolar disorder. She had been on a roller coaster with her moods for years without understanding why. A lack of understanding is common among those who suffer from bipolar disorder. There are several forms of bipolar disorder.

BIPOLAR I DISORDER

Previously known as manic-depressive illness or just manic-depression, this condition is diagnosed in people who have at least one episode of mania. Most people with bipolar I also have major depressive episodes, but these episodes are not required for the diagnosis to be made. Bipolar disorder is equally common in men and women, and occurs in approximately 3 percent of the population. The first episode occurs on average at age 25, but it can occur as early as childhood or later in life. Bipolar disorder has a strong genetic component and is a chronic condition that requires lifelong treatment.

Central to the diagnosis of bipolar disorder is the occurrence of manic episodes. When someone is manic, she talks faster than usual, is more active, and tends to have more confidence. She may have an elated mood, or instead may be more irritable. Often she has an increased sex drive, and she may become sexually promiscuous when that would never be her behavior if she weren't having a manic episode. She may also engage in other reckless behaviors, such as spending money that she does not have. She may stay up all night but still have plenty of energy the next day. She may describe the sensation that her thoughts are racing. The state of mania can feel enjoyable if the mood is elated, but it often causes difficulties at work or with social relationships and can be destructive. She may develop psychotic symptoms, such as hallucinations and delusions, and may require hospitalization.

The criteria for a manic episode according to the *DSM-5* are a distinct period of at least one week (less time if it is determined that the person must be hospitalized because of her symptoms) with an abnormally elevated, expansive, or irritable mood and increased activity or energy plus three or more of the following symptoms (four if the mood is only irritable):

- Inflated self-esteem or grandiosity
- Decreased need for sleep (for example, the person feels rested after only three hours of sleep)
- Excessive talking or pressure to keep talking
- Subjective experience that thoughts are racing
- Distractibility (attention is easily drawn to unimportant or irrelevant external stimuli)
- Increase in activity (socially, at work, or sexually) or psychomotor agitation
- Excessive involvement in pleasurable activities that have a high potential for painful consequences (such as spending sprees, sexual indiscretions, or foolish business investments)

BIPOLAR II DISORDER

Bipolar II disorder is more subtle and may be difficult for you or your doctor to recognize. It consists of one or more episodes of major depression along with at least one episode of *hypomania*. Hypomania is a milder version of mania in which the person can still function fairly normally, sometimes at high levels. During hypomanic periods, the person's mood may be elevated, expansive, or irritable. A hypomanic episode is defined as at least four consecutive days in which the person has three of more of the following symptoms (four if the mood is only irritable):

- Inflated self-esteem (feeling as if she could do much more than she usually could do)
- Decreased need for sleep
- Increased talkativeness
- Feeling that her thoughts are racing
- Distractibility (difficulty sustaining attention)

- Increased activity
- Reckless behavior

This form of bipolar disorder occurs more frequently in women than in men. Hypomanic episodes are not severe enough to cause marked impairment in functioning or require hospitalization, but are noticeable to others and represent a clear change in behavior.

OTHER VARIATIONS

Cyclothymic disorder refers to a chronic, fluctuating mood disturbance in which numerous periods with mild depression and mild hypomanic symptoms occur, without ever developing into full-blown mania or major depression.

Women who have bipolar disorder are more likely than men to have depressive or *mixed episodes*. A mixed episode is one in which manic and depressive symptoms coexist. Mixed episodes have some features of both a manic and a depressive episode, and occur almost every day for at least a one-week period.

Women are also three times more at risk for *rapid cycling*, in which four or more mood episodes occur within a year. This is an unstable and unpleasant state, with mood swings like a roller coaster. Treatment with an antidepressant can precipitate rapid cycling in some people or push them into a manic episode if they have bipolar disorder.

Pregnancy and the postpartum period are especially challenging for women with bipolar disorder. Mood stabilizing medications have potential damaging effects on the baby and must be used with care. Women with bipolar disorder are also at high risk after childbirth of developing postpartum depression or psychosis.

Overall, bipolar disorder is difficult to diagnose. Often the correct diagnosis is revealed only after treatment with an antidepressant for depression precipitates a manic episode. Typically the first episode that a woman with bipolar disorder may experience will be a depression, so that neither she nor her doctors realize that she has this disorder when her treatment is first begun. Anyone being treated for depression with an antidepressant should be watched closely for the emergence of manic symptoms, since this may be the first time that the mania is uncovered.

What Can You Do If You Have Bipolar Disorder?

GET A THOROUGH PSYCHIATRIC INTERVIEW

If you suspect you might have bipolar disorder, or if you have mood swings that you cannot control and want help for them, you should seek a comprehensive psychiatric evaluation. It is easy to miss the diagnosis of bipolar disorder, especially in the setting of primary care. The diagnosis is based primarily on history, because there is no objective measure such as a blood test.

TRY MOOD-STABILIZING MEDICATION

Mood-stabilizing medications are key to the treatment of bipolar disorder (see table 7). Mood stabilizers include lithium salts, derived from the natural element lithium, as well as a number of anticonvulsant medications that have been discovered to be effective for mood management. Lithium is generally believed to be the most effective treatment, but it has limitations due to its side effects. Side effects include possible weight gain and sedation. More importantly, kidney and thyroid function can be affected. The other medications listed in table 7 are anticonvulsants, and they have a variety of possible side effects, including sedation, dizziness, and nausea.

The mood stabilizers vary in their ability to prevent depression; the medication lamotrigine is more effective than lithium or valproic acid in preventing depression. Your doctor can monitor blood levels of some of the mood stabilizers (lithium, valproic acid, and carbamazepine) to verify that the dose is adequate.

Patients I have been treating for years tell me that episodes of mania and depression have been controlled by their medications, which help them maintain a stable mood. Adequate treatment with a mood stabilizer can prevent such episodes from recurring and can give you a sense of stability in your life. You can

TABLE 7 *Mood-Stabilizing Medications*

Brand name	Generic name	Recommended dose range*
Eskalith, Eskalith CR	lithium	900–1,200 mg/day[†]
Depakote	valproic acid/valproate	1,200–1,500 mg/day[‡]
Lamictal	lamotrigine	100–200 mg/day[§]
Tegretol	carbamazepine	400–1,200 mg/day
Trileptal	oxcarbazepine	1,200–2,400 mg/day

*As of 2015.

[†]Lithium should be given in divided doses and the patient's blood levels should be monitored for safety and effectiveness.

[‡]Depakote comes in several forms and can be given once a day (ER version) or in divided doses. The patient's blood levels should be monitored.

[§]Lamictal should be started at 25 mg/day and the dose gradually increased to reduce risk of a rare dangerous rash that develops in some people taking this drug.

also learn to recognize the onset of an episode of either depression or mania, and your doctor can adjust your medications to restore a normal mood.

CONSIDER ANTIPSYCHOTIC MEDICATION

A group of medications known as the antipsychotics can also help stabilize mood. The medications in table 8 are used to treat people who have bipolar disorder as well as people who have psychotic disorders.

Antipsychotic medications have other side effects that should be considered. Thorazine is an older medication that has the risk of causing movement disorder symptoms including tardive dyskinesia, a potentially irreversible neurological condition that produces movements of the mouth and tongue. It can also lead to stiffness, tremors, and jerking movements, which can be controlled with treatment.

The other antipsychotic medications in table 8 are called *atypical antipsychotics* and were developed more recently. Several of the atypical antipsychotics have been given FDA approval for the treatment of bipolar depression: Seroquel (quetiapine), Latuda

TABLE 8 *Antipsychotic Medications Used as Mood Stabilizers*

Brand name	Generic name	Recommended dose range*
Abilify	aripiprazole	15–30 mg/day
Geodon	ziprasidone	80–160 mg/day in divided doses
Latuda	lurasidone	20–80 mg/day
Risperdal	risperidone	2–8 mg/day
Seroquel	quetiapine	300–800 mg/day
Symbyax	olanzapine/fluoxetine	6–12 mg olanzapine/25–50 mg day fluoxetine
Thorazine	chlorpromazine	200–800 mg/day
Zyprexa	olanzapine	10–20 mg/day

*As of 2015.

(lurasidone), and Symbyax (which includes both olanzapine and fluoxetine). These medications are also considered to be mood stabilizers and may be given to bipolar patients who are depressed without precipitating mania.

The side effects of this group of medications include the risks of causing diabetes, weight gain, and the metabolic syndrome (which includes elevated blood pressure, glucose, triglycerides, and cholesterol). These atypical antipsychotic medications have less risk for causing tardive dyskinesia compared to the older, more traditional, antipsychotics (of which Thorazine is the only one listed in the table), but there is still a risk.

Another rare but dangerous side effect of antipsychotic medications is the neuroleptic malignant syndrome. This is a potentially lethal reaction that includes muscle rigidity, fever, changes in blood pressure, and confusion. This condition is considered a medical emergency but can be successfully treated.

Anyone treated with an atypical antipsychotic should be carefully monitored for changes in weight and for possible development of diabetes or increase in lipids. Although these are serious potential side effects, these medications can have much benefit for controlling the mood swings of bipolar disorder.

BEWARE OF ANTIDEPRESSANT MEDICATION

There is controversy among psychiatrists about the best use of antidepressants in people with bipolar disorder, but the general consensus is that they should be added to a mood-stabilizing medication only when needed. If an antidepressant is added, it is advisable to do so only after a mood stabilizer has already been given and is at a therapeutic dose.

Despite what we know about the dangers of giving antidepressant medications to someone with bipolar disorder, many women with this condition are prescribed antidepressant medications. All the antidepressants have the potential to push you into becoming manic or developing rapid cycling. If you are already on a mood-stabilizing medication at a therapeutic dose, and if you continue to have severe depressive symptoms, you might benefit from an antidepressant. You and your doctor will need to watch closely for the appearance of any symptoms of mania, which can develop rapidly. You might ask someone close to you to observe, too, because people with mania do not always recognize it in themselves.

ENSURE ADEQUATE SLEEP

Changes in sleep can herald the onset of an episode of depression or mania, and getting adequate sleep is an important preventative measure for both. Lack of sleep can trigger a manic episode. With depression, sleep may be increased or decreased from normal, and changed sleep is a common symptom. See chapter 6 for a discussion of sleep hygiene, as well as information on various prescription and over-the-counter medications that can aid in sleep. There are a number of strategies that can help you to sleep better, and if you have bipolar disorder it is especially important that you pay attention to your sleep.

SEEK THERAPY

Women with bipolar disorder can benefit tremendously from therapy. For one thing, it will help you to accept and understand this condition. If you can recognize the symptoms of mania when they are mild, you can potentially get help right away and "nip in the bud" a further episode. Similarly, if you feel that you are becoming depressed you can take action to improve your mood. Gaining insight into this disorder, acknowledging that you have it, and learning to recognize the early symptoms of episodes can be immensely helpful.

It is common for women with bipolar disorder to resist this diagnosis. The feelings of mania and hypomania may be enjoyable, and many people do not want to give up this euphoria. Many people choose instead to discontinue their mood-stabilizing medication, which perpetuates the emotional roller coaster. Often patients will tell me that they do not like the idea of taking medication for this disorder. An analogy that I use is that I am sure diabetics wish they did not have to take insulin, but the insulin can help them to lead a healthy life.

One benefit of therapy is that negative thoughts during depression can be addressed with the cognitive approach. Therapy alone is usually not sufficient for those who have bipolar disorder, however. You will likely need to be maintained indefinitely on medications that can help to prevent you from having more episodes as well as being treated when you become depressed or manic again.

PLAN AHEAD WHEN CONSIDERING PREGNANCY

If you have bipolar disorder, you should consider carefully when and whether you want to have children. Untreated bipolar disorder can affect both you and your baby. If you become ill (manic or depressed) during pregnancy, you are more at risk for substance abuse, neglect of your prenatal care, poor judgment, inadequate nutrition, reckless behavior, self-harm, and suicide (in the case of depression).

If you do get pregnant, you need to be aware that treatment has special risks during pregnancy. Most of the mood stabilizers can affect your baby in the womb. One serious risk with mood stabilizers is the danger of birth defects. Specifically, valproic acid and carbamazepine can cause neural tube defects, which are serious birth abnormalities such as spina bifida. Lithium has a small risk of causing cardiac defects. Many pregnancies are unplanned, but for a woman of childbearing age living with bipolar disorder it is wise to think ahead and be cautious when choosing a mood stabilizer. The atypical antipsychotic mood stabilizers have not been available as long as these other treatments, so there is less information about their safety in pregnancy. Ideally you would talk to your doctor about your desire to become pregnant, and this desire would influence the choice of mood stabilizer.

If you stop your medication before you become pregnant, you have a higher risk of a relapse. If you have only had one episode of mania and have been relatively stable, you may be able to taper off your medication and avoid exposure for your baby, especially during your first trimester. If you are treated with a medication during pregnancy, your doctor should use the minimum effective dose and try to use only one medication. You may need to be seen by your doctor more frequently while pregnant.

The postpartum period—the period after giving birth—is also a time of increased risk for you if you are bipolar. You are more likely to develop postpartum depression, and might even develop postpartum psychosis. The latter is a very serious condition in which you may lose touch with reality, develop hallucinations, and sometimes have thoughts of harming yourself and/or your baby. Prepare for this period by discussing your risks and your treatment plan with your doctor.

AVOID STRESS

Women with bipolar disorder are especially vulnerable to stress. Episodes of depression and mania often occur in response to a stressful event. Stay on your medication, avoid alcohol and drugs, and seek ways to maintain your balance, as discussed in previous chapters. Look for what makes you feel calmer, and try to avoid situations that create distress. Cultivate healthy friendships and spend time with positive people. Pay attention to your mood and let your doctor know if you sense you are developing an episode of depression or mania.

If you sense that you are becoming depressed, push yourself to become more active and resist the urge to withdraw from others. Conversely, if you sense that you are becoming manic, limit your activities and seek ways to stay calm.

•

Bipolar disorder is an illness in which periods of depression and mania may occur. The periods of mania can feel good at the time but can cause much destruction. Bipolar disorder can be difficult to recognize, so it is important to seek a thorough evaluation if you suspect that you might have this disorder. There are treatments that can help you to achieve stability, and to lead a more satisfying life without the roller coaster ride of severe mood swings.

RECOMMENDED RESOURCES

BOOKS

Janelle M. Caponigra, MA, Erica H. Lee, MA, Sheri L. Johnson, PhD, and Ann M. Kring, PhD. *Bipolar Disorder: A Guide for the Newly Diagnosed.* Oakland CA: New Harbinger Publications, 2012.

Julie A. Fast and John D. Preston, PsyD. *Loving Someone with Bipolar Disorder: Understanding and Helping Your Partner.* Oakland CA: New Harbinger Publications, 2012.

Kay R. Jamison, PhD. *An Unquiet Mind.* New York: Random House, Inc., 1995.

David J. Miklowitz, PhD. *The Bipolar Disorder Survival Guide: What You and Your Family Need to Know,* 2nd edition. New York: Guilford Press, 2010.

Francis Mark Mondimore, MD. *Bipolar Disorder: A Guide for Patients and Families,* 3rd edition. Baltimore: Johns Hopkins University Press, 2014.

Stephanie McMurrich Roberts, PhD, Louisa Grandin Sylvia, PhD, and Noreen A. Reilly-Harrington, PhD. *The Bipolar II Disorder Workbook: Managing Recurring Depression, Hypomania, and Anxiety.* Oakland, CA: New Harbinger Publications, 2013.

WEBSITES

For Depression and Bipolar Support Alliance (DBSA): www.dbsalliance.org
Website includes educational information and support group
contacts, including both local chapters and online support groups.
For National Alliance for the Mentally Ill (NAMI): www.nami.org
National Institute of Mental Health: www.nimh.nih.gov
Website includes educational information on bipolar disorder.

CHAPTER 10

Women and Grief

I arrived home that summer afternoon puzzled about why my husband was in bed. Had he returned home sick from work? Had he stayed home sick? When I realized that he was dead I was in total shock. He had not been ill and we were planning a vacation in a few days. We were in a very happy stage of our lives.

In the days and weeks that followed, I experienced what so many other widows go through. I had waves of intense sadness as I grieved for the loss of my beloved husband. Yet, I also felt the comfort of being strongly supported by family and friends, and got pleasure from happy memories. I was able to retain my hope for the future, although it was hard to imagine living the rest of my life without my husband. I was able to return to my job and continue to function despite my loss. This was a painful time for me but very different from my earlier experience of depression.

What to Expect When You Are Grieving

Grief touches us all. Loss of loved ones is a universal human experience, yet it remains poorly understood by most people. It can be frightening, and it is hard to know what is "normal." Grief is not unique to women, of course, but since we tend to live longer than men, we are more at risk for the loss of a loved one and over the course of our lives we are more likely to face grief.

Our society does not teach us much about how to grieve. We may find ourselves confused about how to act and feel when we experience a loss. One of the best descriptions I have heard is that bereavement can feel like a personal earthquake, shaking the foundations of a person's life. It can seem so overwhelming and intense that you may wonder at times if you are losing your mind.

Various stages of grief have been described. Elisabeth Kübler-Ross, a Swiss American psychiatrist, introduced a model for understanding the dying process in her 1969 book, *On Death and Dying*. According to Kübler-Ross, the stages of grief are denial, anger, bargaining, depression, and acceptance. These stages may not occur in sequence and may be felt simultaneously. Her model has been applied to the dying person as well as to the survivors.

Denial refers to the disbelief that occurs immediately after suffering a loss. When someone is in the stage of denial, the loss that has just occurred seems unreal. They may feel as if they are in a fog, or on autopilot. They may not be able to feel their own sadness, but instead go through the motions of doing what must be done for the funeral and afterwards. They may say that they feel fine and may not yet feel the gravity of the loss that has occurred. Denial is one of our defense mechanisms, a psychological protection against losses too painful to accept. This is usually a temporary stage that resolves quickly and rarely does someone become stuck in the denial phase.

Anger is described as the second stage, in which the griever may feel resentment, envy, or rage toward self or others. The feelings are out of proportion to the situation and are unusual for her. This anger can be irrational, and may be expressed by irritability and short-tempered reactions to everyday frustrations. She may experience considerable resentment toward others whom she considers insensitive. She may also experience resentment toward those whom she feels are responsible for the loss, such as the doctors who failed to communicate adequately, to diagnose soon enough, or to find a treatment that was effective. Anger can also occur toward the deceased on many levels. It is common to have anger about being left behind by the loved one. It is easy for the bereaved to take out their anger on those who are closest to them, and it is helpful to remember that this behavior is temporary and is common in the grief process.

Some types of death provoke much more anger. Suicide is one of the most difficult losses to resolve, and typically a person feels a mixture of emotions. Anger, self-blame, confusion, disbelief are mixed together with the sadness that would occur after any loss. Homicide can also cause an understandable level of anger and rage. It may be difficult to resolve feelings about a homicide until there is some sense that justice has been served to the perpetrator; on the other hand, some people find comfort only when they manage to forgive the perpetrator.

Bargaining is the third stage, and refers to a common phenomenon of trying to persuade God or a higher power to reverse the loss. This stage was identified by Kübler-Ross in the context of patients who were dying and desperately seeking a way to postpone their own death. They may have promised to reform their lifestyle, for example, if only they could have more time with their loved ones. It is common for the family members of the terminally ill to attempt to bargain with God.

Depression is the fourth stage of the grief process defined by Kübler-Ross. At this stage, the reality of the loss becomes unavoidable. The sadness may feel unbearable at times and it may be hard to find solace. At times one who is grieving may cry inconsolably, or find it hard to envision happy times again in the future. It may seem hopeless to go on.

Acceptance is the final stage described by Kübler-Ross. Some losses, such as an unexpected death of a child, are harder to accept than others. Yet over time, the unthinkable becomes part of your life narrative. The pain of your loss may never be fully gone, but it feels different over time. You can regain your ability to enjoy life as you accept the reality of your loss.

Grief is a painful but necessary process that has much in common with depression. If you are grieving, you may have changes in your sleep and appetite. You may feel fatigued, lose your usual interests, and have difficulty concentrating. You may feel as if you are in a "fog." You may also feel fear and anxiety along with your sadness. Physical symptoms such as aches and pains are also common during grief.

In contrast with depression, grief has a different pattern and course. Those who grieve typically experience "waves" of sadness, sometimes triggered by reminders of the deceased. The sadness is less continuous than with depression. Those who grieve are usually able to continue functioning and do not develop thoughts of suicide. Over time, the grief becomes less intense and joy in life can return. The amount of time needed for that improvement to occur varies widely.

Another difference between grief and depression is how it is understood. Most psychiatrists and mental health professionals would *not* try to "fix" someone's pain of grief. You need to experience your grief in order to overcome it, scary and painful as that may be. You may need to learn to allow yourself to grieve, rather than to try to avoid it. There is a time and place for using medications to help those people who have depression and anxiety, but acute grief is something that needs to be experienced in order for healing to occur. After a loss, there are no shortcuts. Seeking quick relief, such as through alcohol or drugs or other behaviors, may only prolong your suffering. Grief must be gone through to get past.

The Role of Anticipatory Grief for the Terminally Ill

Anticipatory grief occurs when you know that someone you love will die soon. It occurs before the death of your loved one and can be similarly painful to the grief felt afterward. The grieving that occurs during the illness may help you to be able to accept the loss when it does occur. This advance knowledge gives time for you and your loved one to say goodbye. There is an opportunity to resolve differences, settle business affairs, and plan for the funeral together. This can be a valuable occasion in your relationship with your loved one.

Death and dying are difficult topics for most people to discuss. We live in a society that avoids the topic of death, and when you have a loved one who is ill you may feel that you are betraying him or her if you discuss it. Some caregivers and patients feel that it is important to never give up, and may have difficulty accepting the reality that we all must die. The inevitability of death may be a concept that is hard to accept in your heart until you have experienced loss.

Conversations about death can be a relief to the dying, as well as to elderly people before their final days. There are choices to be made (for example, does the person want to be buried or cremated?), and there may be special requests about the funeral. In a larger sense, talks at this time may take on a level of poignancy that is rarely experienced in life. Petty resentments may dissolve, forgiveness may be given between loved ones, and wishes for the future and final messages can be expressed. In some cases, however, personal and family tensions may increase. The dying person may reject his or her death, or long-held resentments between family members may surface.

If family members avoid the topic of death, it can be difficult for them to make decisions about life-prolonging medical procedures. Families may try to hold on to their loved one even after the likelihood of recovery becomes dim. Now that hospitals routinely ask patients whether they have documented their wishes in advance directives and living wills, this topic is more directly addressed in the medical setting. Families may benefit from taking a straightforward approach as well and seize opportunities for important discussions.

Hospice programs provide a valuable service for the terminally ill as well as for their families. I highly recommend that you ask your doctor to refer you to hospice services if you or your loved one is facing the end of life. Hospice offers a variety of services including nursing and palliative care, counseling, ministry, and friendship. Hospice staff can help families overcome their reluctance to talk about death and can increase their understanding of the dying process.

As I was writing this book, my father was declining from metastatic cancer and ultimately he passed away. On several of my visits, I met his hospice volunteer, Jimmy. My father introduced Jimmy as his "best friend." The two of them often would watch football games together, and my father confided in him about his life. In my eulogy at the funeral I thanked Jimmy for his loving support of my father. The minister responded with encouragement for those present to be like my father and keep making new friends until their last days, something that is quite possible when interacting with hospice staff. Hospice is a wonderful organization full of warm and caring people who are familiar with the dying process and able to guide the dying and their families through this experience. They helped my father and my family tremendously.

What Is "Complicated Grief"?

Many who grieve seek guidance on what they should do to resolve their grief. They may worry about what is "normal." Grief is a painful and potentially overwhelming experience, and there are no clear road maps. Some people get stuck in their grief and are unable to move on with their lives.

Complicated grief is now called persistent complex bereavement disorder in DSM-5, and it is the term used to describe grief that is not resolved normally after 12 months. Signs that your grief may be complicated include:

- Continued sense of disbelief regarding the death
- Unresolved anger and bitterness over the death
- Intense yearning and longing for the deceased
- Preoccupation with thoughts of the loved one, often including disturbing thoughts related to the death itself
- Withdrawal and avoidance, including steering clear of situations and people that are reminders of the loss

Complicated grief needs to be distinguished from major depression (discussed in chapter 6). Some key differences are:

- The sadness of grief is primarily associated with missing the deceased, rather than being a pervasive gloom

- With grief, interest in memories of the deceased is maintained, including longing and yearning for contact as well as pleasurable reveries
- In grief, feelings of guilt are focused on interactions with the deceased, rather than being more pervasive, as in depression
- Grief may include being preoccupied with positive experiences with the deceased, rather than on past failures and perceived misdeeds

In short, depression encompasses your whole life, while grief is focused on the loss of a loved one.

Complicated grief also needs to be differentiated from post-traumatic stress disorder (discussed in chapter 7). Some of the distinctions are:

- PTSD is triggered by a physical threat rather than the loss that triggers grief
- The primary emotion of PTSD is fear instead of the sadness felt in grief
- Nightmares are common in PTSD but rare with grief
- Painful reminders of PTSD are linked to the traumatic event itself; the painful reminders with grief are more pervasive and unexpected
- Finally, grief can include pleasurable remembrances as well as yearning and longing for the deceased, whereas PTSD involves purely negative memories and sensations

A sign that you may be stuck in your unresolved grief is constantly replaying the events surrounding the death of your loved one. You may retell the story of what happened when you see friends and family. You may relive the experience in your mind and continue to despair.

Some losses are much more difficult to resolve. Suicide often devastates family and friends. After a suicide, it is common to have a mixture of emotions including anger, guilt, and sadness. Survivors frequently blame themselves for not seeing signs that the person was about to kill herself and taking action to prevent it. They may have intense anger that the deceased made the choice to leave this world and abandon the family. The consequences of suicide by a loved one can last for many years or a lifetime. Support groups for survivors of suicide as well as individual therapy may be very helpful. Learning that others struggle with the same emotions can be healing.

Homicide is another loss that is especially difficult to resolve. Rage at the killer is common and can greatly complicate the grief process. Legal proceedings about the death, which can last for months or years, may revive grief feelings again and again. Resolution of grief may feel impossible until the perpetrator has been identified and punished. Forgiveness may feel impossible but can for some people be healing. If other family members are suspected in the death, that intensifies the emotional process even further and may lead to much anguish.

Death of a child is an overwhelming loss for most people. No parent wants to bury her child. Regardless of the age of the child, this loss brings with it many layers of disappointment and pain. Many dreams will be unfulfilled. Guilt about the death is common, as is anger toward others who might have prevented the death. Some couples divorce after they lose a child, after their marriage is ripped apart by mutual blame or by their individual difficulties in working through their grief.

How Can You Tell If You Are Developing Depression After a Loss?

Differentiating between grief and major depression can be difficult, and there is no clear consensus in psychiatry or psychology about how to make this distinction. Currently there is a debate underway about the length of time that is "normal" for someone to experience bereavement before it should be considered major depression, but time is not the primary determinant of whether your grief has turned into depression.

You might be developing depression after a loss if you exhibit any of the following symptoms:

- Inability to function (some amount of decreased functioning is expected with grief, but with depression you may feel unable to get out of bed, go to work, or take care of yourself)
- Loss of your capacity to experience pleasure or your interests (you may no longer feel joy in any situation)
- Suicidal thoughts
- Preoccupation with self-criticisms and feelings of worthlessness
- Feelings of guilt other than about the events of the death itself
- Hallucinations, such as hearing voices or seeing things, that persist after the initial period of grieving
- Excessively long duration of the grieving process

This last criterion is the trickiest one. How long is too long to grieve for a loved one? What should you expect? When should you worry about yourself and consider seeking help?

Those who have experienced losses know that it is not unusual to have symptoms of grief for six or twelve months, or even longer, but the symptoms are usually episodic rather than continuous. They continue to appear as waves of sadness, and over time the waves become less frequent. The potential to experience pleasure returns despite the grief. Some individuals feel that they should continue to mourn for prolonged periods as part of a spiritual tradition, or even as a member of a support group. In some cultures it is appropriate to have an extended period of mourning.

The key factor in judging the "expected" duration of grief is how severe your symptoms are. Some periodic sadness and tearfulness about your loss is likely to go on for the rest of your life, especially when you encounter poignant reminders of your loved one; this is nothing to be feared or avoided. The trigger could be a song that you shared or one that reminds you of the deceased. It could be the celebration of a holiday or family event without your loved one present, or the anniversary of important days such as birthdays. What makes us human is our capacity to love another, and we feel sad when we lose someone we love. The duration is worrisome only if you have severe symptoms that persist over time.

The DSM-5 allows for the possibility that someone may have major depression in conjunction with grief, occurring as soon as two weeks after a loss. Most people who have a loss will not develop major depression. Normal grief is a healthy reaction to a loss, consisting of "waves" of emotions that include sadness and also pleasant memories. Major depression can develop after a variety of stressors and losses, but is more continuous and severe than healthy grief.

There Are Many Varieties of Grief

We ought not judge others based on how much or how little they mourn. Each of us is unique in our grieving. Some people will cry a lot more than we do if that is their temperament. Others may not easily be observed to be crying at all. They may not feel comfortable letting others see them cry or let others know how they are dealing with their loss. That is okay! The number of public tears shed has no bearing on how much the person is grieving or how much love was there for the person who died.

Some may judge widows and widowers for how quickly they choose to remarry. When is "too soon" for a widowed person to "date" or to consider remarriage? I have heard stories of people who were in a new relationship or even remarried days or weeks after they lost their spouse. Dating that quickly may be done as a "rebound," and it may be healthier to learn to live more independently before entering a new relationship. Nevertheless, I urge caution in making such judgments about what other people do in their personal lives.

Some may judge other family members, especially children, for how well they support the widow or widower. I would consider the individual needs of each family member. We all grieve in different ways and it is easier for some people to talk about their feelings and to reach out to others. The widow and widower are not the only ones who are feeling the loss. Friends, siblings, parents, children, other family may all be affected by a death. I think it is much more productive to focus on gratitude for the support people offer rather than think about what support was not offered.

The community of widows is worldwide. Strangers can become an important source of comfort if they are able to truly empathize with your loss. At many times in life, it is our kindness to one another that bonds us and gives hope.

Cultures vary greatly in their rituals for mourning and for honoring the dead. Even within one country there are big differences. Racial, ethnic, religious, and cultural diversity results in a variety of outward expressions of grief. Many traditions include wearing black clothes and exhibiting quiet, respectful behavior. Some mourners may leave a room untouched, or create a zone of the home with many photographs and memorabilia. There is nothing wrong with creating such a memorial to your loved one. The challenge is to focus on your loss but not let it dominate your life.

In some traditions, many days or weeks are spent in mourning. In Thailand there is no mourning period; people just continue their normal routines. The Jewish tradition includes seven days of shiva, in which the community comes to comfort the mourners, and the month following the death is also considered a special time of mourning. In contrast, many workplaces in the United States give three days of bereavement leave (if that), which greatly underestimates the time that will be needed. It is important to allow yourself time to honor your loss and to receive support from others. Healing cannot be rushed.

How Can You Grieve Well and Go On Living?

LEARN WHAT TO EXPECT

It will not always hurt as severely as it does in the beginning. Talk to others who have been through similar losses. It is common to feel overwhelmed, confused, frightened, and angry. You may relive the events surrounding the death over and over. You may need to tell your story multiple times.

Part of the difficulty of handling a major loss is that there are so many decisions to be made at a time when you may feel unable to think clearly. Some choices cannot be put off—for example, you must make decisions in short order about the funeral itself—but many others can likely wait. It may help you to get a list from your funeral home of the short-term tasks to be done, such as whom to notify. Beware of making major decisions when you have just suffered a big loss. For most people, it is better to wait, possibly even a year, before considering major changes such as switching jobs, selling your house, or starting a new relationship. Give yourself time. You may think quite differently about your decisions a year from now.

ALLOW YOURSELF TO FEEL SAD

Many people are frightened when they cry or feel very sad. They may think that they are "having a meltdown." The intensity of emotions that can be unleashed after a major loss can surprise you. Do not be scared by your sadness. Grief is a necessary part of being human. It is all a matter of degree. Occasional crying spells do not mean that you are losing control or losing your mind.

Others may feel unable to cry, and this may cause worry too. Accept your feelings as they come, and give yourself permission to feel them without second-guessing yourself.

HONOR THE MEMORY OF YOUR LOVED ONE

After the funeral, you may still feel the need to pay tribute to your loved one. There are both private and public ways to convey recognition. You may want to have a very private ritual, such as lighting candles at special times or you may want to find ways to share your memories with others. You may be better able to move on with your life if you take the time to create a special memorial such as a window, statue, or other tribute to your loved one.

FOCUS ON YOUR SPIRITUALITY

The death of a loved one might prompt you to focus and clarify the priorities in life. If you are part of a spiritual community, you may want to rely on the group for support and to immerse yourself in your own spirituality. You may want to read scripture and to discuss your thoughts with your faith leader or with friends who are similarly spiritual. The spiritual community may provide organized support resources. If you do not have a spiritual community or a clear spiritual identity, this may be a time for you to explore your faith. You may find that you are more receptive to spiritual discussions and experiences than in the past.

The loss of your loved one may challenge your faith. Some people respond with anger and bitterness and turn away from God. They may be unable to accept their loss and become overwhelmed with protest and rage for some time. Author Elizabeth Brown discusses her own spiritual journey in her book, *Surviving the Loss of a Child.* She describes a turning point after the death of her daughter in which she reconciled the tragedy of her loss with the blessings of her own survival. She was able to strengthen her faith as she turned to God for guidance. She developed more empathy for others in their losses and found that life took on a deeper meaning.

REQUEST HOSPICE SERVICES

Hospice is a beautiful organization with the ability to help those who are dying and their families understand and accept the process with grace. If you are grieving in anticipation of a loss, or dealing with your own dying process, ask your doctor to refer you to a local hospice service. In addition to providing care of the terminally ill, hospice also offers support for their families. Medicare and other insurance plans pay for hospice services, including most pharmaceuticals, medical equipment, twenty-four hour/seven days a week access to care, and support for the family after a death. Hospice volunteers can provide much personal attention and encouragement.

ALLOW YOURSELF TO ACCEPT SUPPORT

In the beginning, you will probably need and want time alone. You should listen to yourself and take the opportunity to experience feelings and recall memories. You may want to look at old photographs and other memorabilia.

As you feel ready, accept invitations. In time you may be inclined to extend yourself to others as well. Push yourself to do things with others. You are likely to feel rewarded for reaching out.

CHOOSE WHERE AND WITH WHOM TO SPEND YOUR TIME

You may find that your feelings shift about whom you want to see and spend time with. For example, you might find that some couples who previously socialized with you and your partner may stir up your sense of loss. You might find yourself enjoying the company of other widows and widowers who know firsthand what you are going through. Alternatively, you might not be ready to identify yourself with other widows and you may want to stay safely within your established social circle.

If you are lucky enough to have friends who are sensitive and compassionate, they will allow you to talk freely about your loss and will help you to enjoy life again. These friends might have also been close to your loved one and may be sharing the loss. Pay attention to your feelings when you are with others, and seek comfort from nurturing relationships.

When you lose your partner, you are suddenly single again. It may have been many years since you were not attached. You might find that you want to spend more time with others who have experienced a similar plunge into the single world. Your journey ahead will be new to you, but others on similar paths can provide understanding and guidance.

GET EXERCISE

Again I recommend exercise as a way to enhance your mood. It may feel easier to withdraw and feel sad, but if you push yourself to be active it can go a long way to improve how you feel physically and emotionally. Many studies have shown both the health benefits and the mood benefits of exercise. Exercise oxygenates your blood and helps your body to release its natural mood elevators, the endorphins. The exercise does not have to be formal and you do not have to use expensive equipment. Simply taking long daily walks can be enough.

WRITE IN A JOURNAL

We often rely on our loved ones as sounding boards to discuss our lives, review daily events, and air concerns and feelings. After the death of a confidant, you are faced with the challenge of learning to stand on your own and provide your own counsel. You also need to find a way to put your loss in perspective with your life narrative.

Writing daily in a journal can help fill this void. In some respects, journaling is a way to become your own best friend. Give yourself time with your journal to reflect at the end of each day. Express your feelings and strive to soothe and encourage yourself as well. Be sure to note the good things that happen in addition to the hurt you may feel.

REVISIT YOUR LOVED ONE IN YOUR IMAGINATION

One practice that may help you with your grief process is to imagine that you are conversing with your loved one about your loss. Picture how your loved one would respond to you. You may also benefit from further imaginary interactions with your loved one as you work through your grief. This may help you to feel his or her continued presence as well as provide a way to work through unresolved issues at the time of the death.

FOCUS ON YOUR OWN LIFE GOALS

Think about what you would like to do with the remainder of your life if your grief were not so intense. Set small daily goals for yourself and gradually move in the direction of your larger goals. If you dream of travel, plan to visit a friend who will be supportive. You may want to sign up for a class to pursue an interest that you have deferred.

As previously mentioned, it may be helpful to avoid making any significant decisions or changes for a year. On the other hand, there is no one right way to go through the grief process. The key concept here is that it is important to allow yourself time to experience grief and recover from it before you make big changes. You may feel very differently about your life and your options later, when your grief is less acute.

BE ALERT TO THE SYMPTOMS OF MAJOR DEPRESSION

As discussed previously, it can be difficult to distinguish between normal bereavement and major depression. Both are characterized by much sadness, changes in sleep and appetite, decreased energy, difficulty concentrating, and reduced interests. Bereavement, especially loss of a partner, can trigger depression. Consider seeking an evaluation from your primary care physician or a psychiatrist if any of the following occur:

- Your grief symptoms are so intense that you cannot continue to function
- You begin to hear voices or see things that are not there, some weeks after the person's death
- You develop suicidal thoughts
- The duration of your grief is excessively long, and you are unable to move on with your life

As noted above, there is no strict definition for the duration of "normal" grief. In general, six to twelve months has been considered an appropriate time to experience the intensity of grief. If you continue to struggle with your feelings of grief after twelve months, or if you develop any suicidal thoughts or are unable to function, it would be wise to seek an evaluation. On the other hand, do not be surprised or alarmed if you continue to have intermittent feelings of grief for years, or possibly for the remainder of your life. Expect that anniversary dates, holidays, birthdays, and other significant family events may cause a return of your sadness. On such occasions you may feel more down without realizing the cause. Take the time to honor your feelings when this occurs.

If you find yourself reliving your pain on a frequent basis many months after the loss, or crying and reexperiencing the trauma, you may benefit from getting some help. Therapy would be a good way to begin. You may also profit from an evaluation for the possible need for medication.

•

Loss is unavoidable, and we all feel grief at some point in our lives. At times the bereavement process can feel overwhelming and bewildering. It is important to allow yourself to grieve, and usually the best way to get past the grief is to go through it. If you find that you are incapacitated by your grief, if you become suicidal, or if your grief persists for an excessively long period, you may benefit from seeking help. Usually time will help you to put your loss into perspective and to move forward with your own life.

RECOMMENDED RESOURCES

BOOKS
George Bonanno, PhD. *The Other Side of Sadness: What the New Science of Bereavement Tells Us about Life After Loss.* New York: Basic Books, 2009.
Joyce Brothers, PhD. *Widowed.* New York: Ballantine Books, 1992.
Elizabeth B. Brown. *Surviving the Loss of a Child: Support for Grieving Parents.* Grand Rapids, MI: Revell, 2010.
Marta Felber. *Finding Your Way After Your Spouse Dies.* Notre Dame, IN: Ave Maria Press, 2000.
Ann K. Finkbeiner. *After the Death of a Child: Living with Loss through the Years.* Baltimore: Johns Hopkins University Press, 1998.

Elisabeth Kübler-Ross, MD. *On Death and Dying.* New York: Simon & Schuster/Touchstone, 1969.

Therese A. Rando, PhD. *How to Go on Living When Someone You Love Dies.* New York: Bantam Books, 1988.

WEBSITE

For GriefShare: www.griefshare.org/ Includes opportunity to enroll to receïve 365 daily e-mails, includes spiritual focus

CONCLUSION

A Woman's Resilience

As women, we face many stresses throughout our lives and we may at times feel that we cannot handle the struggle. I hope that within these pages you have found useful suggestions for understanding your moods and how stress and other factors influence you. It is so easy to neglect our own emotional health, especially when we are often busy caring for others. We all need to slow down at times and increase our efforts to care for ourselves. As they say on airplanes, we need to put on our own oxygen masks before we can help others.

Resilience is a concept that has become popular in recent years and refers to the ability to rebound after experiencing stress. Why is it that some people can undergo adversity and bounce back even stronger, while others become overwhelmed? What makes some people more adaptable than others, more able to be positive despite the hardships of life?

The relatively new branch of studies called positive psychology focuses on what helps people to do well and be healthy rather than emphasizing what constitutes illness. A number of books on this topic are available and are included at the end of this chapter. I have also listed a recent documentary called *Happy*, which discusses choices each of us can make that will promote our own happiness.

We cannot control what happens to us, and we certainly cannot control other people in our lives. But we can choose our reactions to life. I hope that you will use the tools within this book and choose healthy behaviors and coping strategies. Life can be much more rewarding when you do!

RECOMMENDED RESOURCES

BOOKS

Martin E. P. Seligman, PhD. *Authentic Happiness: Using the New Positive Psychology to Realize Your Potential for Lasting Fulfillment.* New York: The Free Press, A Division of Simon & Schuster, 2003.

Martin E. P. Seligman, PhD. *Learned Optimism: How to Change Your Mind and Your Life.* New York: The Free Press, a Division of Simon & Schuster, 2006.

MOVIE

Happy. Documentary by Roko Belic, 2011 (available from Public Broadcasting Service and on Netflix).

BIBLIOGRAPHY

American College of Obstetricians and Gynecologists Committee on Health Care for Underserved Women (2012).Opinion No. 524: Opioid abuse, dependence, and addiction in pregnancy. *Obstetrics & Gynecology* 119:1070–76.

American Psychiatric Association (2013). *Diagnostic and Statistical Manual of Mental Disorders*, 5th edition (DSM-5). Washington, DC: American Psychiatric Publishing.

Blechman E. A. and Brownell K. D., eds. (1998). *Behavioral Medicine and Women: A Comprehensive Handbook*. New York: Guilford Press.

Castle D. J., Kulkarni J., and Abel K. M., eds. (2006). *Mood and Anxiety Disorders in Women*. New York: Cambridge University Press.

Chambers C. D., Hernandez-Diaz S., Van Marter L. J., et al. (2006). Selective serotonin-reuptake inhibitors and risk of persistent pulmonary hypertension of the newborn. *New England Journal of Medicine* 354 (6): 579–87.

Frank E., ed. (2000). *Gender and Its Effects on Psychopathology*. Washington, DC: American Psychiatric Publishing.

Friedman R. A. (2012). Grief, depression, and the DSM-5. *New England Journal of Medicine* 366: 1855–57.

Gold J. H. and Severino S. K., eds. (1994). *Premenstrual Dysphorias: Myths and Realities*. Washington, DC: American Psychiatric Publishing.

Grigoriadis S., VonderPorten E. H., Mamisashvili L., et al. (2014). Prenatal exposure to antidepressants and persistent pulmonary hypertension of the newborn: Systematic review and meta-analysis. *BMJ* 348:f6932.

Hales R. E., Yudofsky S. C., and Roberts L. W. (2014). *The American Psychiatric Publishing Textbook of Psychiatry*, 6th edition. Washington, DC: American Psychiatric Publishing.

Herrin M. (2003). *Nutritional Counseling in the Treatment of Eating Disorders*. New York: Brunner-Routledge.

Jensvold M. F., Halbreich U., and Hamilton J. A., eds. (1996). *Psychopharmacology and Women: Sex, Gender, and Hormones.* Washington, DC: American Psychiatric Publishing.

Jones H. E., Kaltenbach K., Heil S. H., et al. (2010). Neonatal abstinence syndrome after methadone or buprenorphine exposure. *New England Journal of Medicine* 363 (24): 2320–31.

Jordan J. V., Kaplan A. G., Miller J. B., et al. (1991). *Women's Growth in Connection.* New York: Guilford Press.

Karasu S. R. and Karasu T. B. (2010). *The Gravity of Weight.* Washington, DC: American Psychiatric Publishing.

Keyes K. M., Cheslack-Postava K., Westhof C., et al. (2013). Association of hormonal contraceptive use with reduced levels of depressive symptoms: A national study of sexually active women in the United States. *American Journal of Epidemiology* 178 (9): 1378–88.

Ko J. Y., Farr S. L., Dietz P. M., and Robbins C. L. (2012). Depression and treatment among U.S. pregnant and nonpregnant women of reproductive age, 2005–2009. *Journal of Women's Health* 21(8): 830–36.

Kornstein S. G. and Clayton A. H., eds. (2002). *Women's Mental Health: A Comprehensive Textbook.* New York: Guilford Press.

Legato M. J. (1997). *Gender-Specific Aspects of Human Biology for the Practicing Physician.* Armonk, NY: Futura Publishing Company.

Leibenluft E., ed. (1999). *Gender Differences in Mood and Anxiety Disorders: From Bench to Bedside.* Washington, DC: American Psychiatric Publishing.

Lewis-Hall F., Williams T. S., Panetta J. A., and Herrera J. M. (2002). *Psychiatric Illness in Women: Emerging Treatments and Research.* Washington, DC: American Psychiatric Publishing.

Lock J., Le Grange D., Agras W. S., and Dare C. (2001). *Treatment Manual for Anorexia Nervosa: A Family-Based Approach.* New York: Guilford Press.

Mehler P. S. and Andersen A. E., eds. (1999). *Eating Disorders: A Guide to Medical Care and Complications.* Baltimore: Johns Hopkins University Press.

Meyer M. C., Johnston A. M., Crocker A. M., and Heil S. H. (2015). Methadone and buprenorphine for opioid dependence during pregnancy: A retrospective cohort study. *Journal of Addiction Medicine* Jan 22 (EPub ahead of print).

Miller J. B. (1976). *Toward a New Psychology of Women.* Boston: Beacon Press.

Miller L. J., ed. (1999) *Postpartum Mood Disorders.* Washington, DC: American Psychiatric Publishing.

Mitchell J. E., Devlin M. J., de Zwaan M., Crow S. J., and Peterson C. B. (2008). *Binge-Eating Disorder: Clinical Foundations and Treatment.* New York: Guilford Press, 2008.

Morrison M. F. (2000). *Hormones, Gender, and the Aging Brain: The Endocrine Basis of Geriatric Psychiatry.* New York: Cambridge University Press.

Rasgon N. L., ed. (2006). *The Effects of Estrogen on Brain Function*. Baltimore: Johns Hopkins University Press.

Reefhuis J., Devine O., Friedman J. M., et al. (2015). Specific SSRIs and birth defects: Bayesian analysis to interpret new data in the context of previous reports. *BMJ* 351:h3190.

Romans S. E. and Seeman M. V., eds. (2006). *Women's Mental Health: A Life Cycle Approach*. New York: Lippincott Williams & Wilkins.

Shear K., Frank E., Houck P. R., and Reynolds C. F. (2005). Treatment of complicated grief: A randomized controlled trial. *Journal of the American Medical Association* 293 (21): 2601–8.

Steiner M. and Koren G., eds. (2003). *Handbook of Female Psychopharmacology*. London: Martin Dunitz.

Steiner M., Yonkers K. A., and Eriksson E., eds. (2000). *Mood Disorders in Women*. London: Martin Dunitz.

Stewart D. E., ed. (2005). *Menopause: A Mental Health Practitioner's Guide*. Washington, DC: American Psychiatric Publishing.

Stewart D. E. and Robinson G. E., eds. (1997). *A Clinician's Guide to Menopause*. Washington, DC: American Psychiatric Publishing.

Stewart D. E. and Stotland N. L., eds. (1993). *Psychological Aspects of Women's Health Care*. Washington, DC: American Psychiatric Publishing.

Teatero M. L., Mazmanian D., Sharma V. (2014). Effects of the menstrual cycle on bipolar disorder. *Bipolar Disorders* 16: 22–36.

Toffol E., Heikinheimo O., Koponen P., et al. (2011). Hormonal contraception and mental health: Results of a population-based study. *Human Reproduction* 26 (11): 3085–93.

Wainrib B. R., ed. (1992) *Gender Issues across the Life Cycle*. New York: Springer Publishing.

Yonkers K. A., Brown C., Pearlstein T. B., et al. (2005). Efficacy of a new low dose oral contraceptive with drospirenone in premenstrual dysphoric disorder. *Obstetrics & Gynecology* 106: 492–501.

Zerbe K. (2008). *Integrated Treatment of Eating Disorders: Beyond the Body Betrayed*. New York: W. W. Norton.

INDEX

abdominal breathing, 136
Abilify (aripiprazole), 119, 165
abortion, 56–57
acupuncture, 37
addictions: causes of, 152–53; and
depression, 98–99, 153–54; and
gender differences, 141; impact of,
in pregnancy, 151; and tolerance,
153; treatment for, 154–58
Addison's disease, 98
adolescence: "acting out" behavior
and, 11, 20; and communication,
20; and cutting, 10, 12; depression
during, 11–13, 22–24; and developmental issues, 10; eating disorders
during, 13–16, 18–20; healthy
activities during, 21; hormonal
changes in, 10; and medications,
21–22; and parenting, 10–11, 20–22;
and relapse prevention, 157–58; and
self-destructive behaviors, 10–11;
stressors during, 10
adoption, 58–60
aging: depression and, 79–83; and end
of life issues, 78–79
agoraphobia, 129
Al-Anon, 155
Alateen, 155
Alcoholics Anonymous (AA), 155,
157
alcoholism, 150–58
alcohol use, and depression, 139
alpha-interferon, 99

alpha-methyldopa, 99
Alzheimer's disease, 98
Ambien (zolpidem), 106
Anafranil (clomipramine), 117,
145–46
Antabuse (disulfiram), 156
antidepressants: approved by FDA for
anxiety disorders, 145; and bipolar
disorder, 119, 166; commonly used,
116; older types of, 117; safety of,
during pregnancy, 48–50; types and
recommended dosages of, 115–17;
use of, in adolescents, 21–22; use of,
in anxiety disorders, 144–48; use of,
while breastfeeding, 54–55; use of,
in depression, 113–20; use of, in
elderly, 83; use of, for premenstrual
syndromes, 37–38
antipsychotics: and the elderly, 83;
use of, in depression, 119; use of, as
mood stabilizers, 164–65
anxiety disorders: anxious depression, 134; body dysmorphic disorder, 133; excoriation (skin picking)
disorder, 133; generalized anxiety
disorder, 126–27; hoarding disorder,
133; obsessive-compulsive disorder, 131–33; panic disorder, 127–29;
posttraumatic stress disorder (PTSD),
134–36; social anxiety disorder (social
phobia), 130–31; specific phobia,
129–30; trichotillomania (hair-pulling
disorder), 133